Getting Ready for My Dentist Visit
Preparing Kids for Better Dental Health

This book belongs to:

Written by Dr. Fei Zheng-Ward   Illustrated by Moch. Fajar Shobaru

Copyright © 2024 Fei Zheng-Ward

All rights reserved. Published by Fei Zheng-Ward, an imprint of FZWbooks. No part of this book may be copied, reproduced, recorded, transmitted, or stored by any means or in any form, electronic or mechanical, without obtaining prior written permission from the copyright owner.

Identifiers: ISBN 979-8-89318-030-5 (eBook)
              ISBN 979-8-89318-031-2 (paperback)
              ISBN 979-8-89318-067-1 (hardcover)

Your teeth help you chew your favorite foods and speak your favorite words, and they give you a beautiful smile.

That's why it is important to take good care of them.

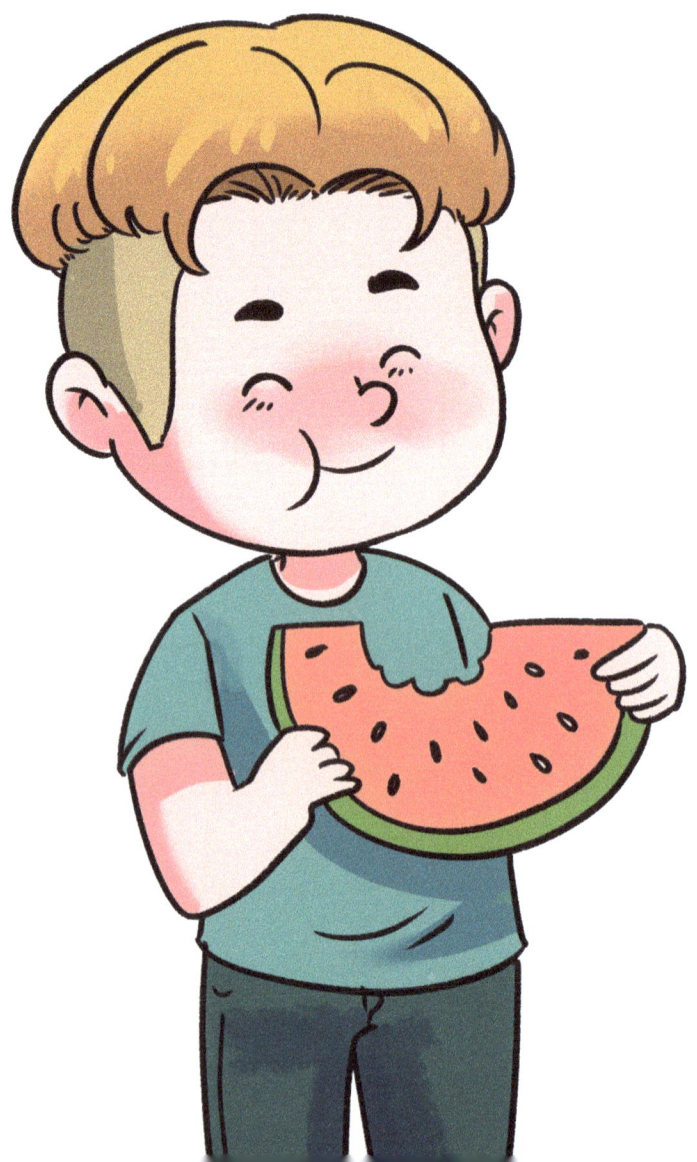

How many teeth do you have?

Write your answer here: _____

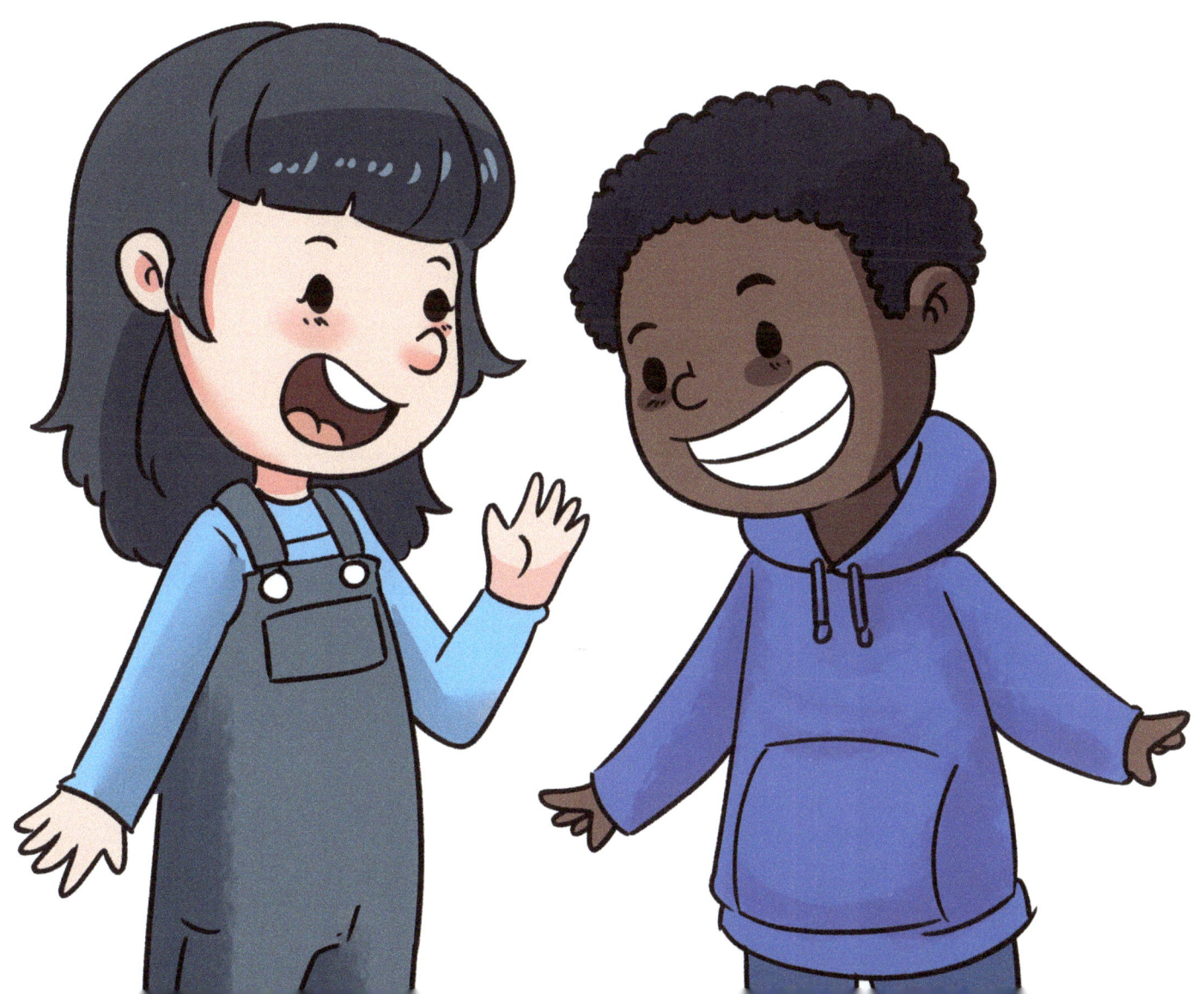

A dentist is a doctor who helps keep teeth and mouths healthy.
Your mom, dad, grandma, and grandpa all go to the dentist.
Did you know that dogs and cats get their teeth checked, too?
And so do zoo animals.

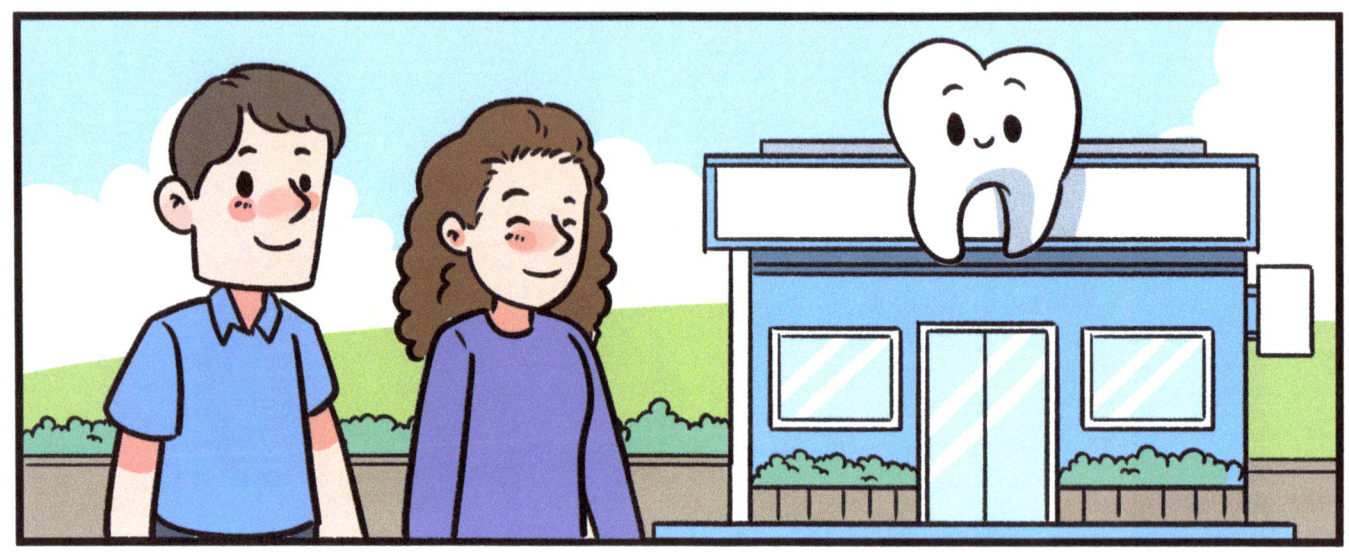

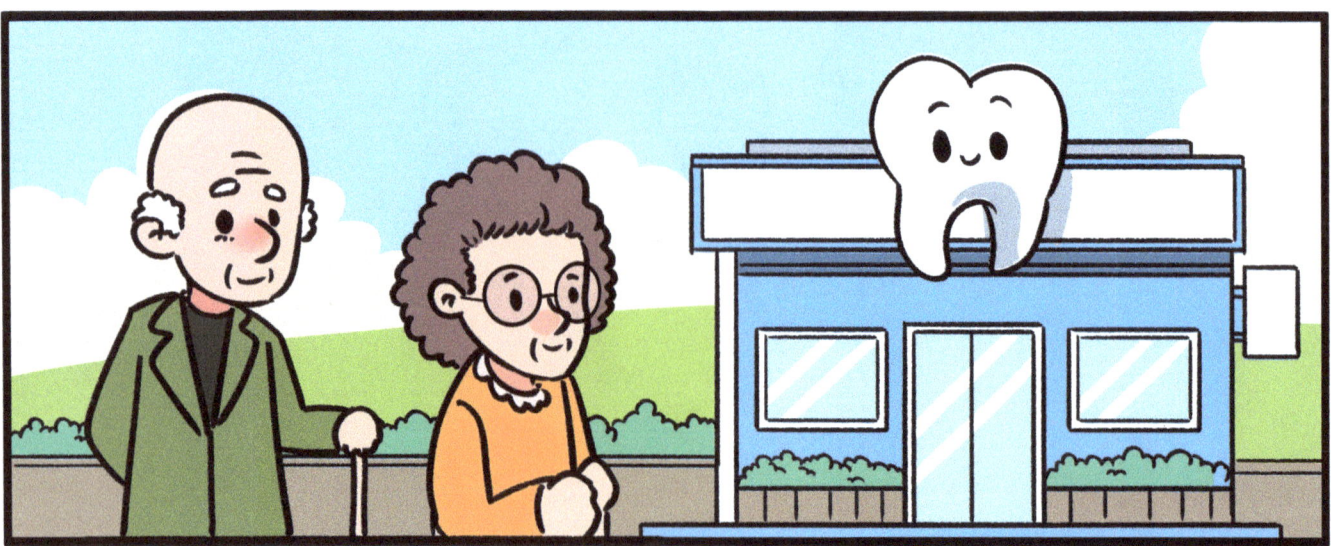

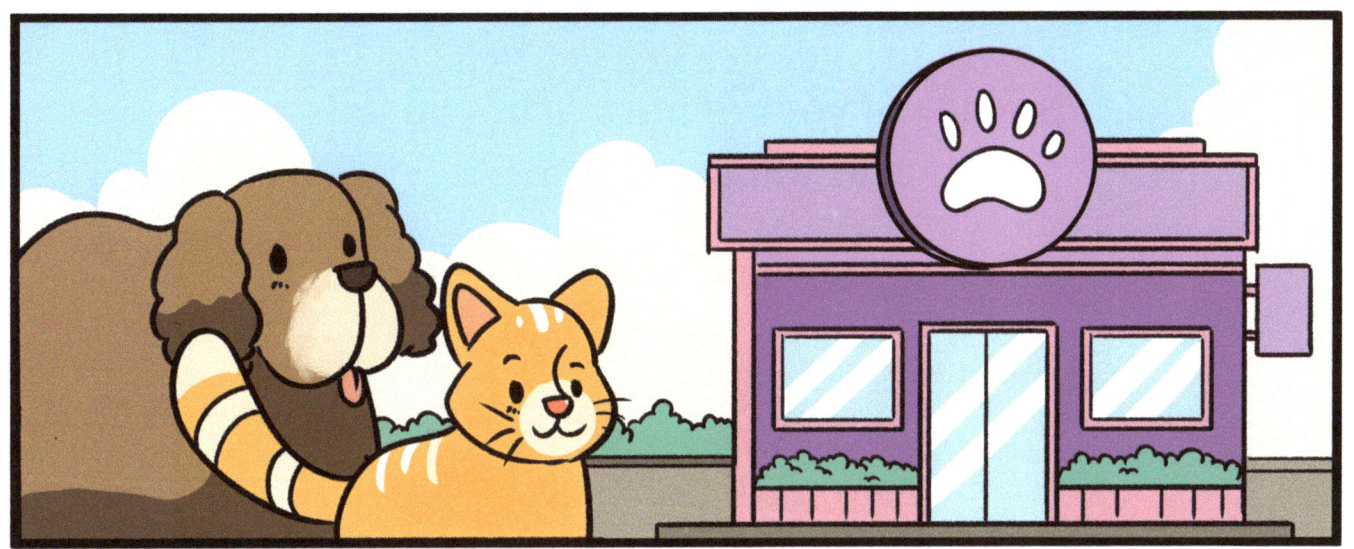

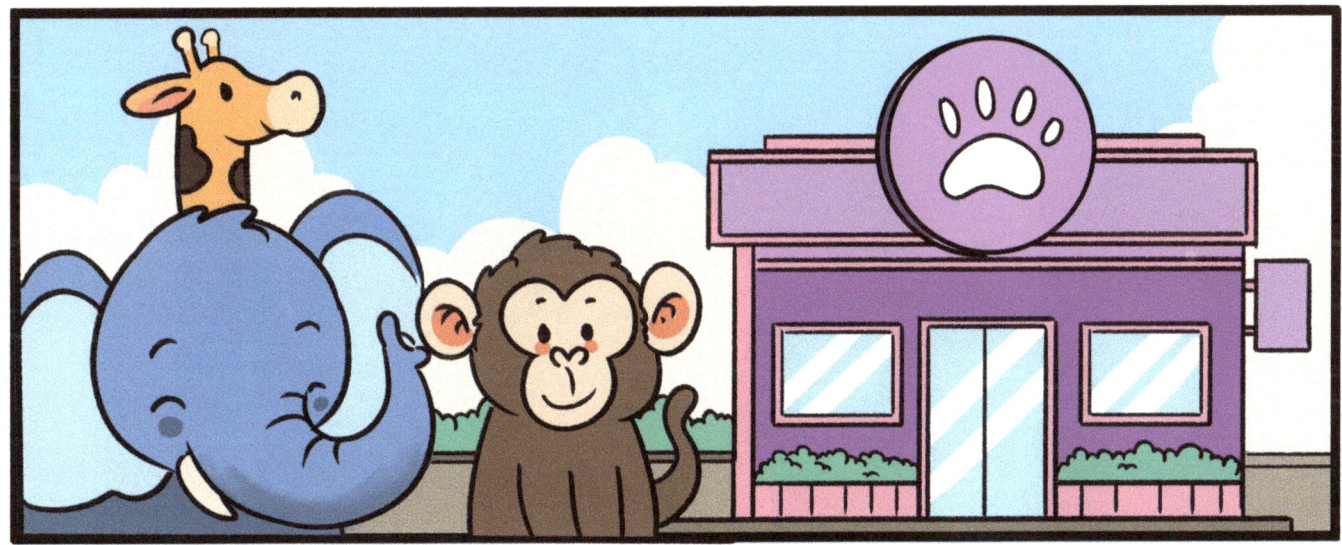

Whether you have 1 tooth or 32 teeth, everyone goes to the dentist.

Have you been to a dentist before?

Circle your answer: Yes   or   No

On the day of your dentist visit, you will arrive at the dental office.

You can bring your favorite toy or blanket.

You may feel a little nervous; that's OK.

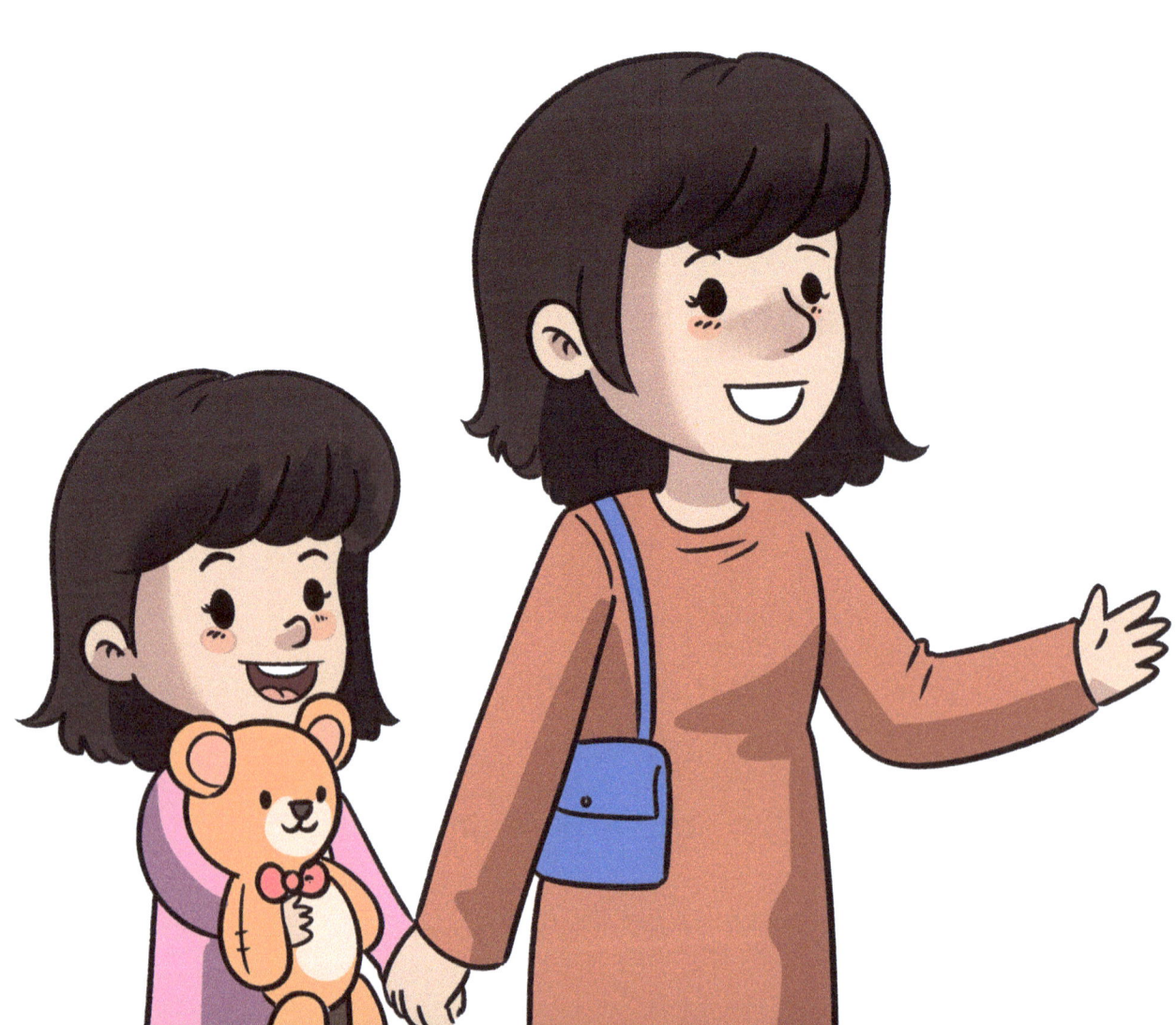

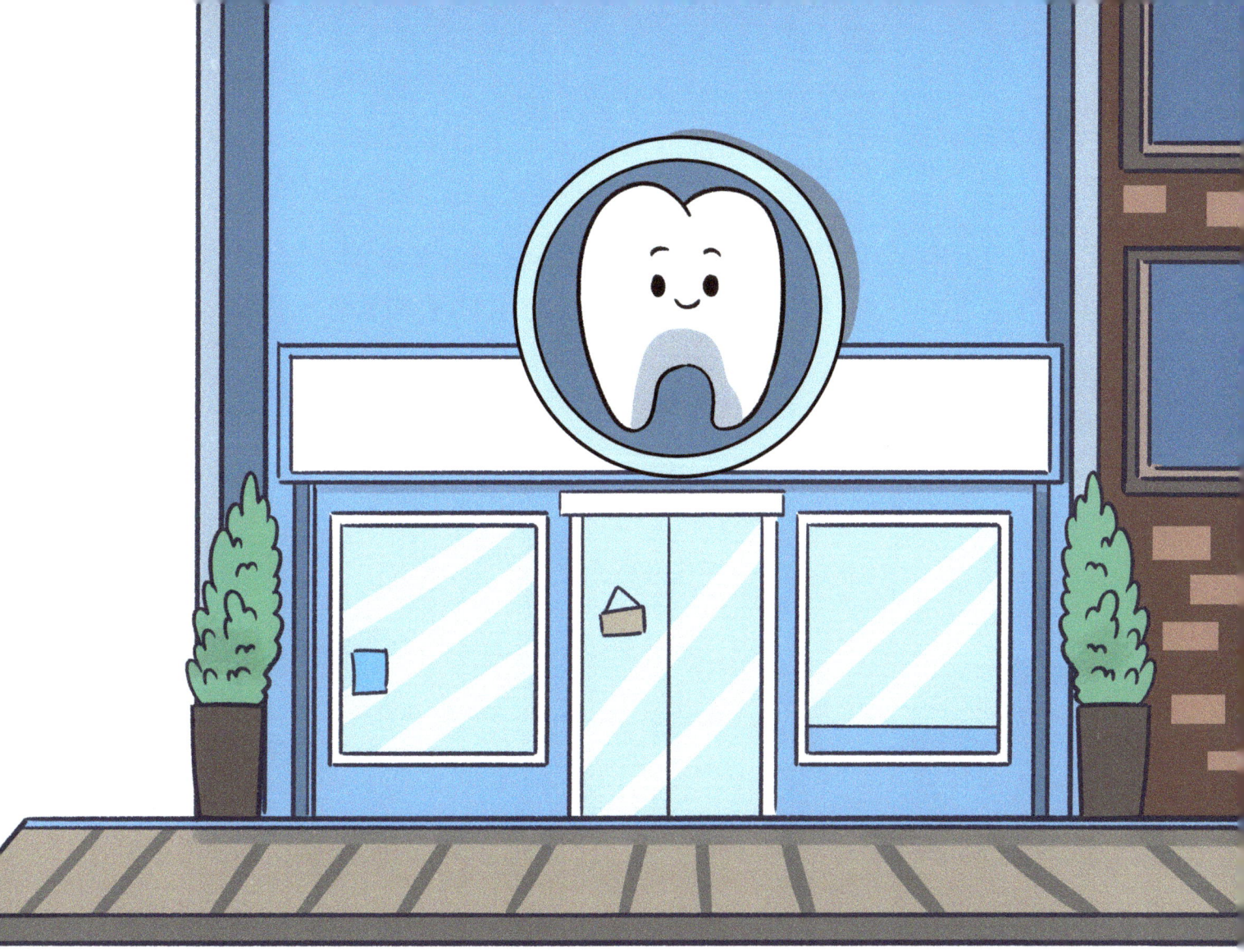

What do you plan to bring with you?

Write your answer here:

_____

You will check in at the front desk and give them your name and birth date.

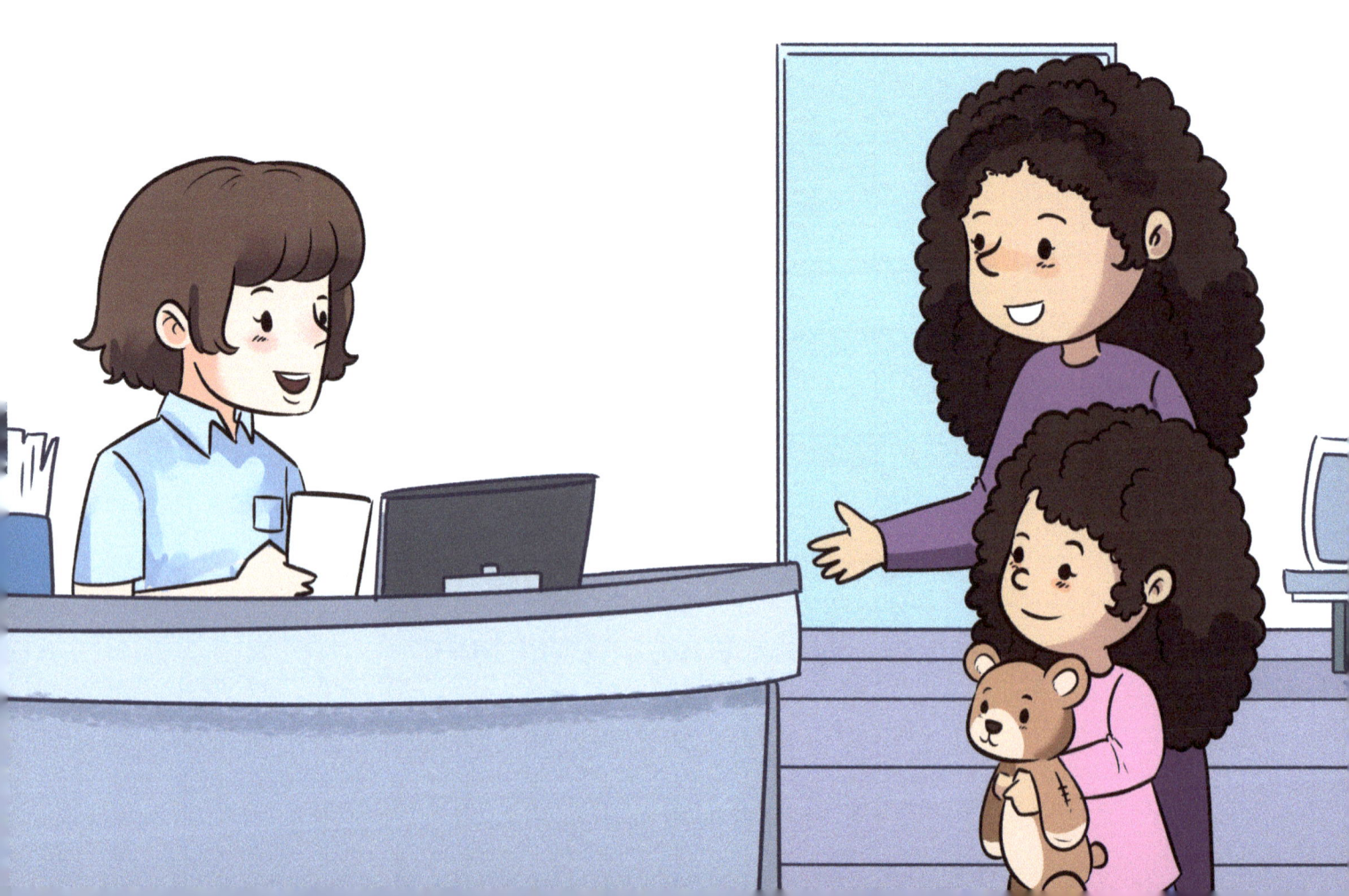

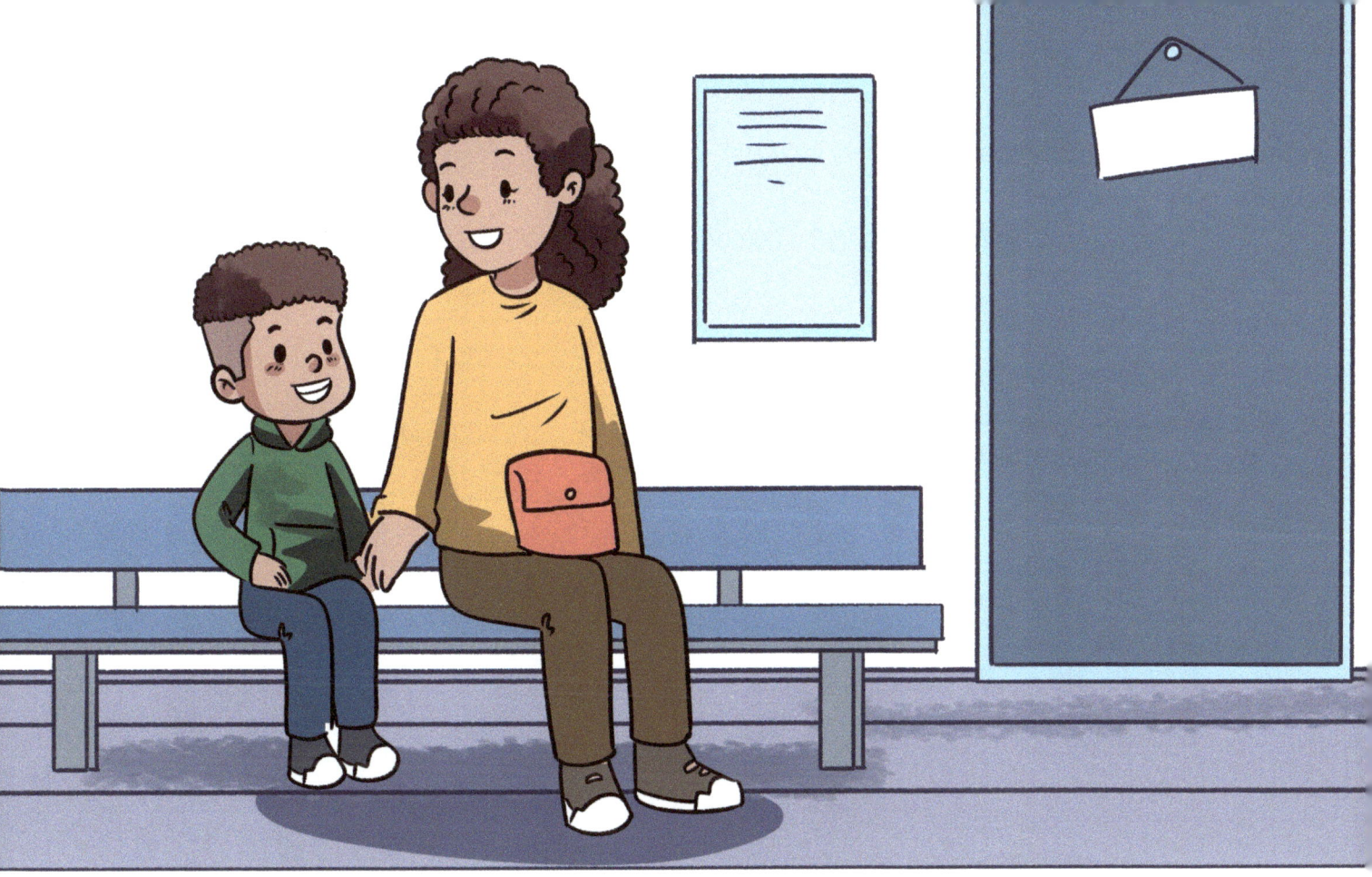

After checking in, you and your parent or guardian will wait in the waiting room until your dentist is ready to see you.

_____, you've got this!
(Write your name above)

Everyone is here to cheer you on!

Let's check out the room they have prepared for you.

Can you spot the following in the room?

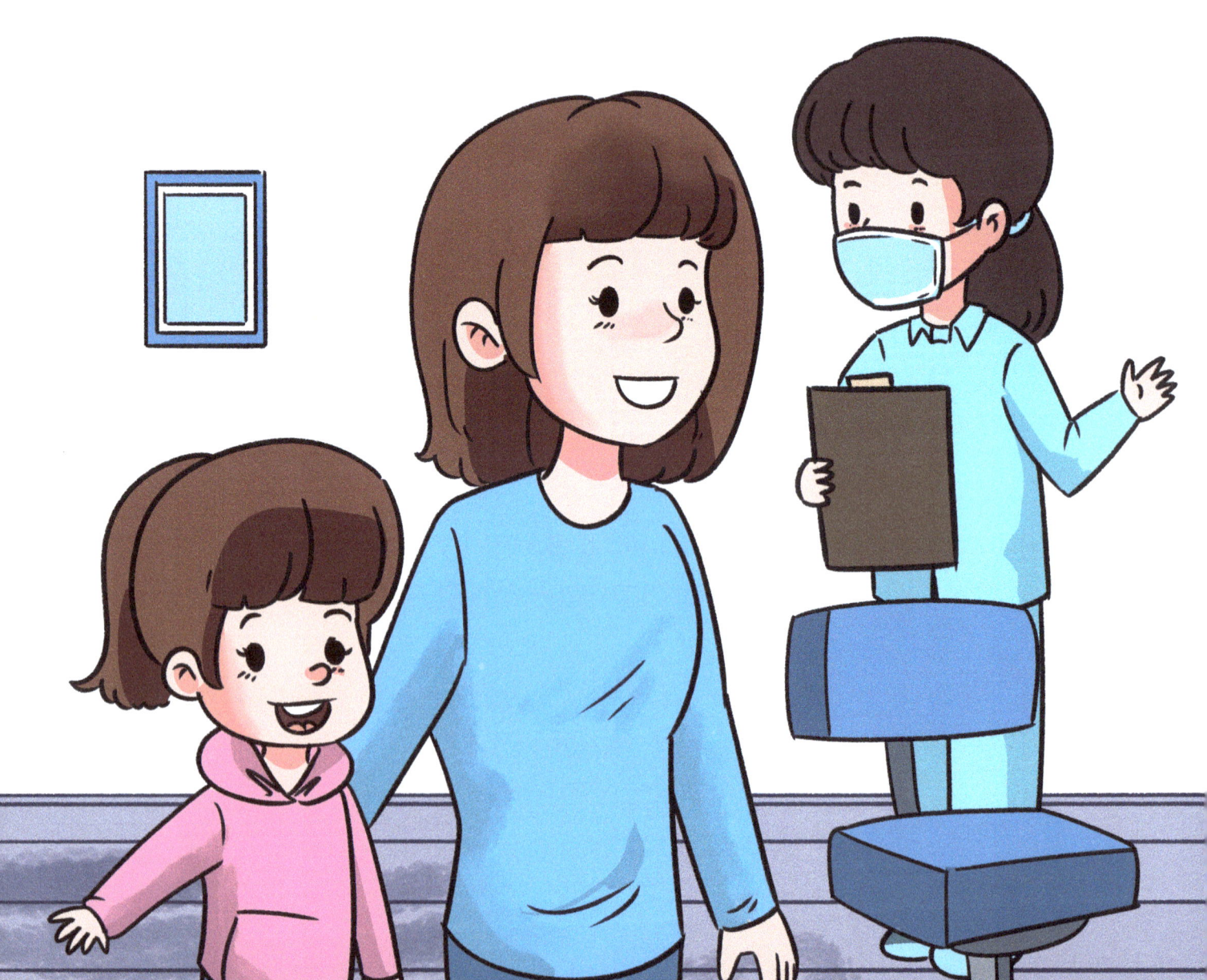

1. A big chair that can move up and down
2. A bright light the dentist uses to see inside your mouth
3. A chair for your parent, guardian, or your favorite toy
4. Your dentist's helper wearing a mask
5. A monitor for you to watch a show while the dentist looks at your teeth

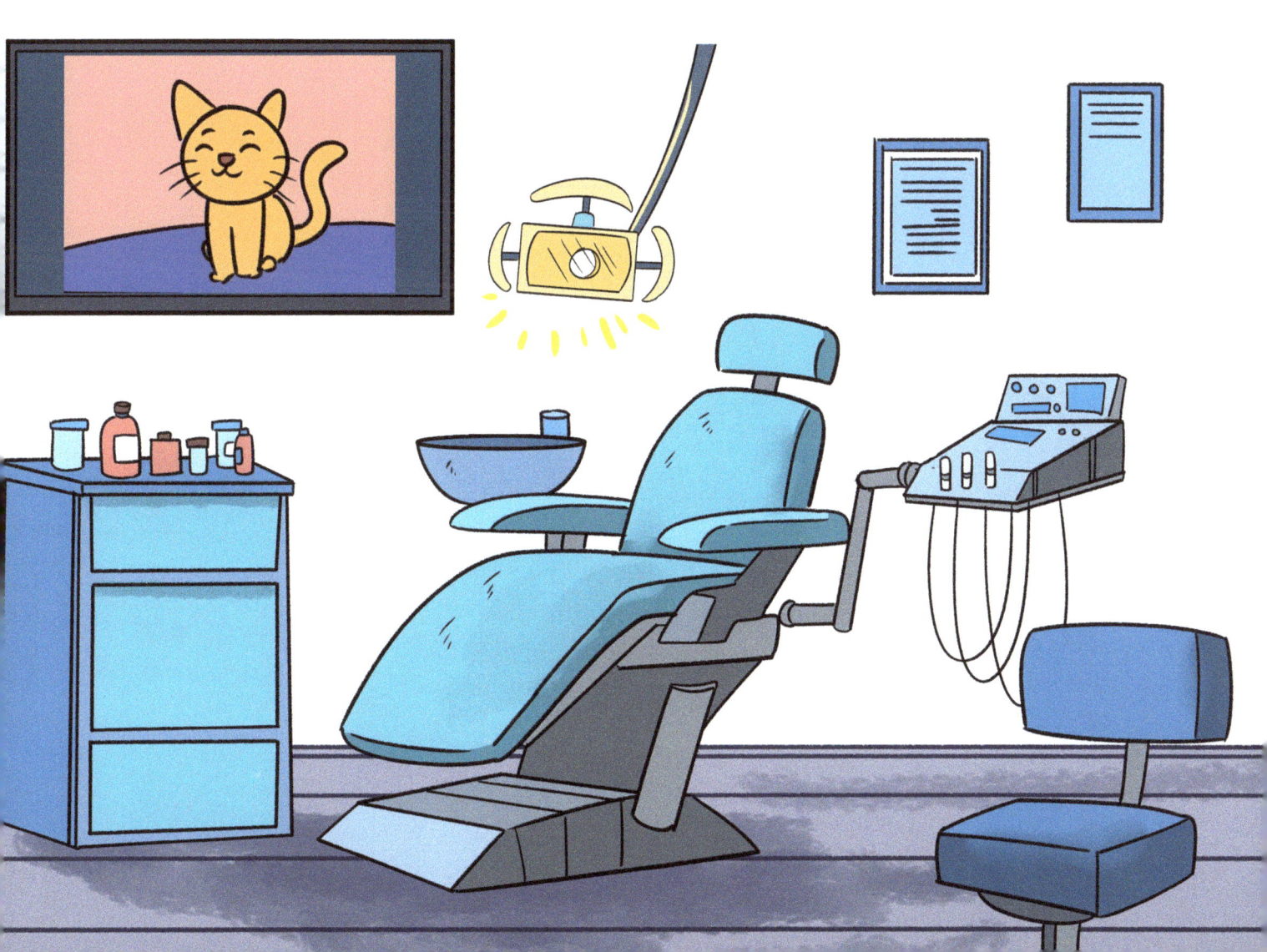

After you get in that special big chair, you may ask if you can go up and down in it.

Cool, right?

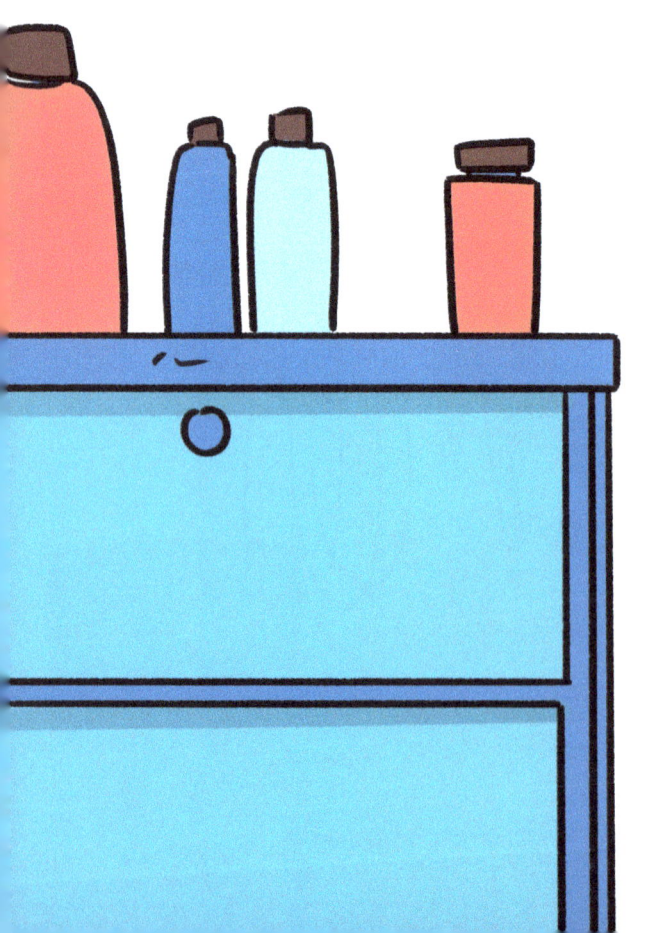
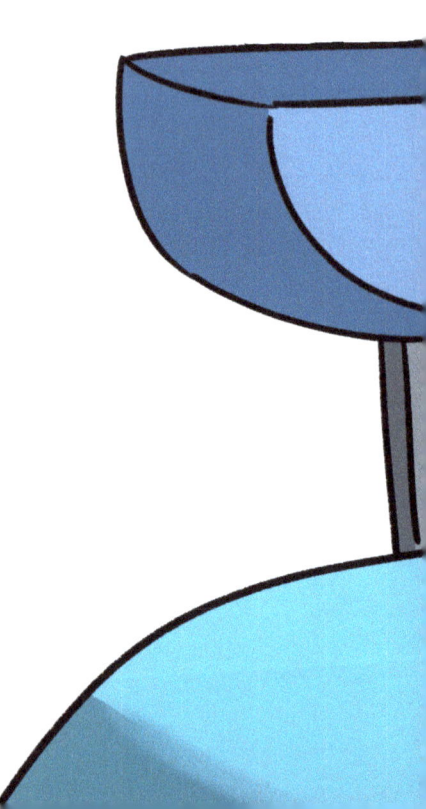

Relax your muscles and lean back in the chair.
It's very comfortable!

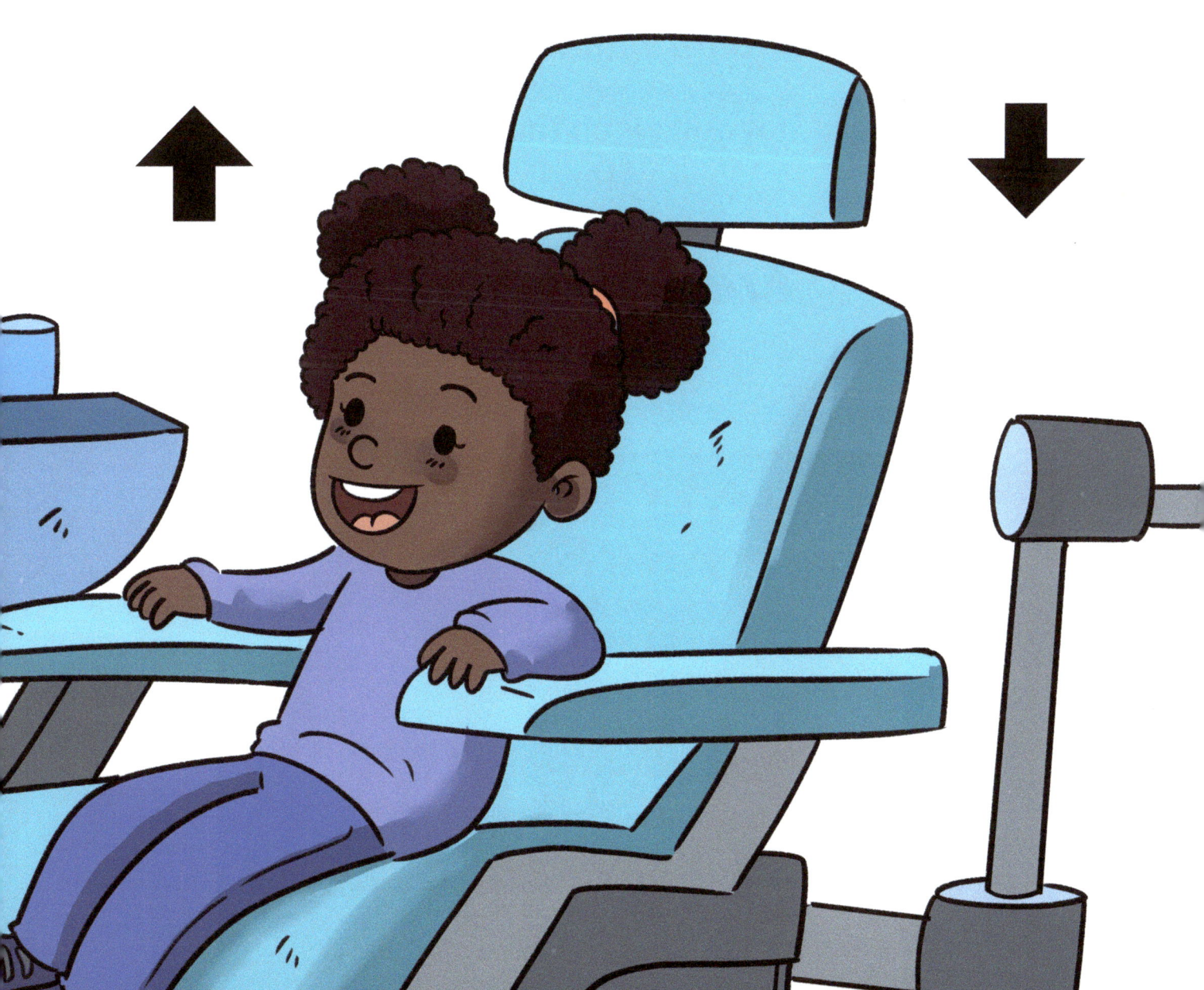

Sometimes, they take x-ray pictures to see the inside of your teeth, how your teeth are growing, and cavities.

You get to wear a big apron for the photo shoot because they don't need pictures of the other parts of your body.

Don't forget to stay still when they're taking pictures of your teeth.

Are you ready?

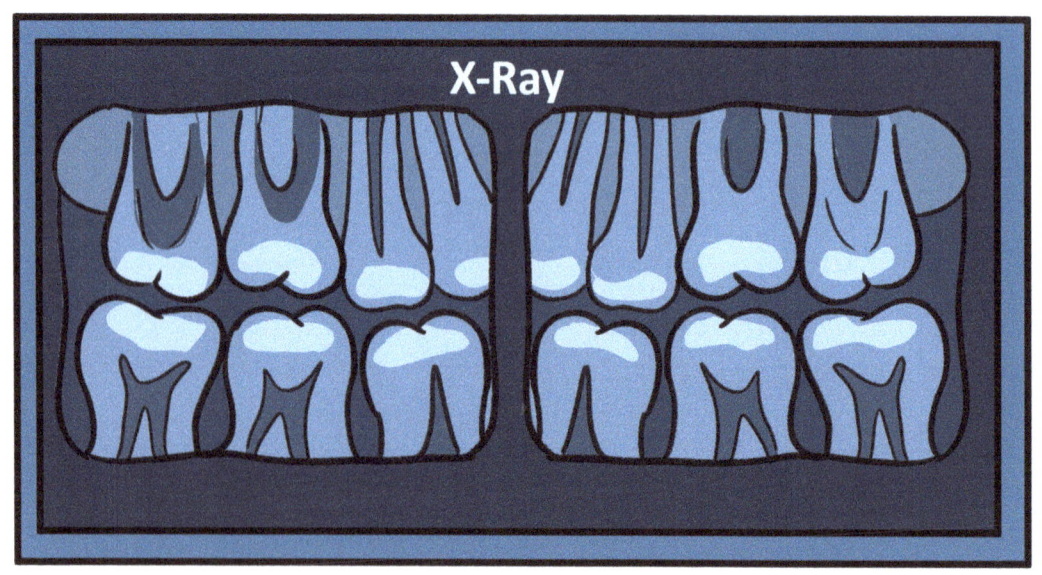

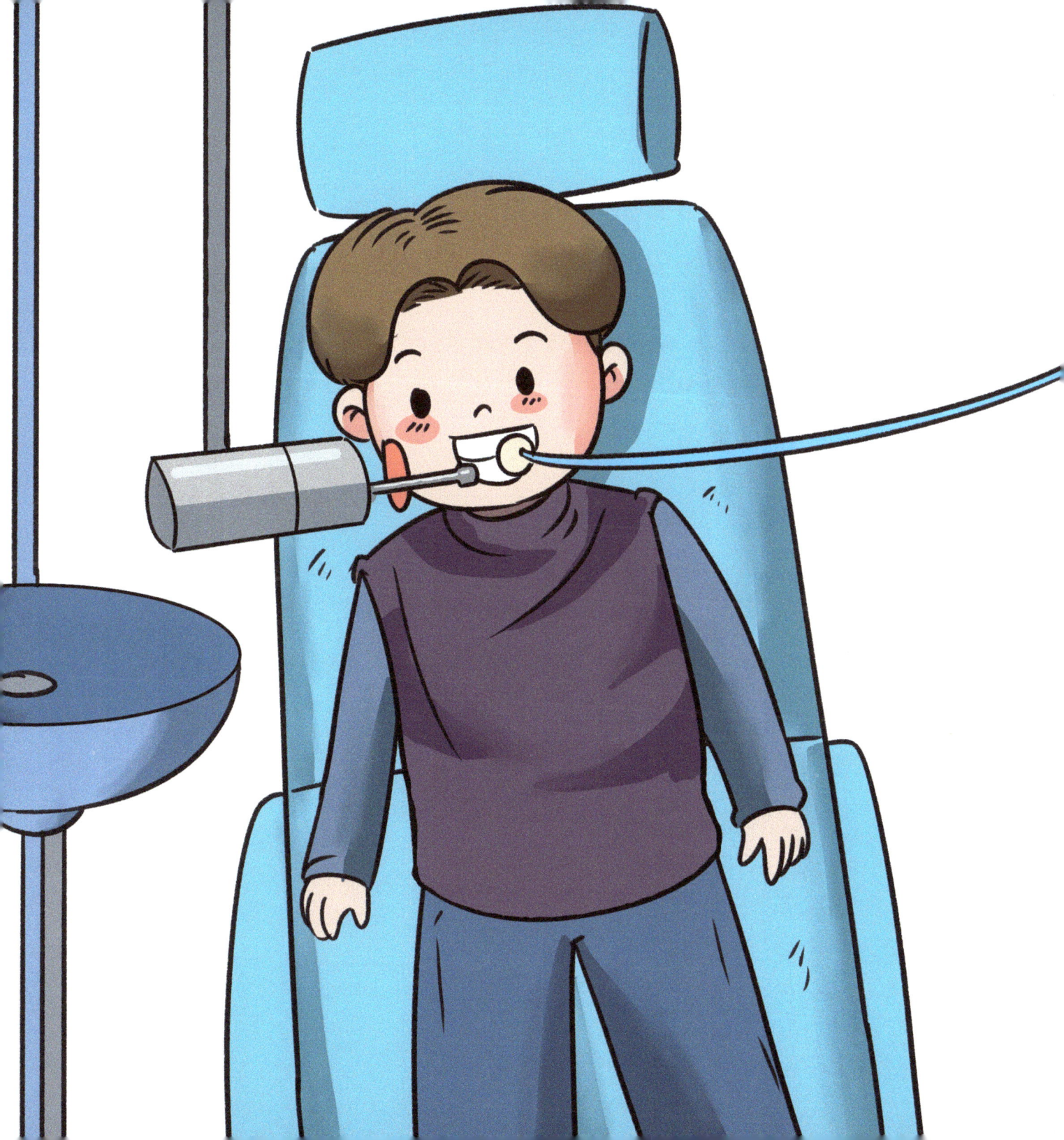

You will get a paper bib before they start cleaning your teeth.

Soon, you will meet your dentist, who's friendly, careful, and gentle.

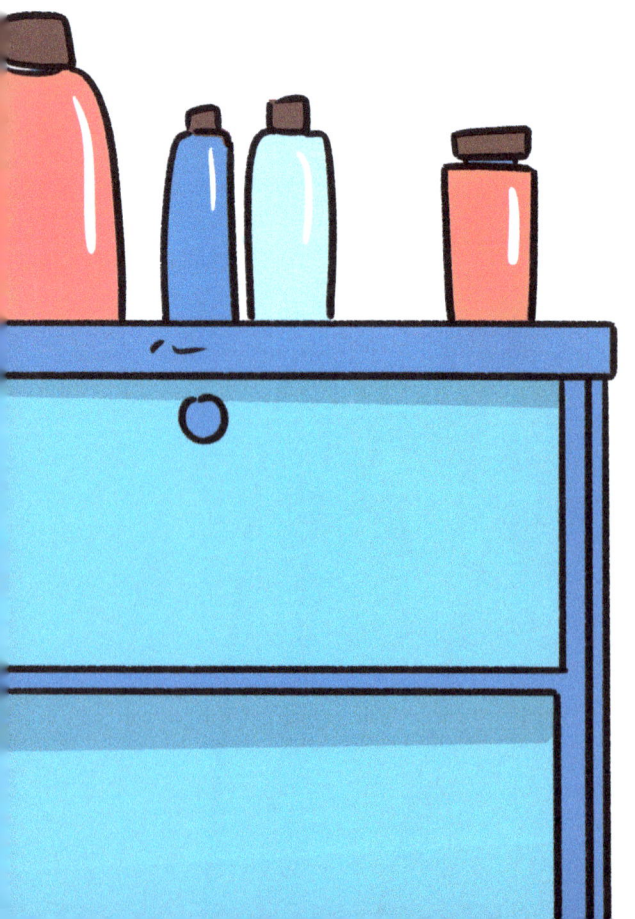

Did you know that your dentist loves to show you their smile, and they would like to see yours, too?

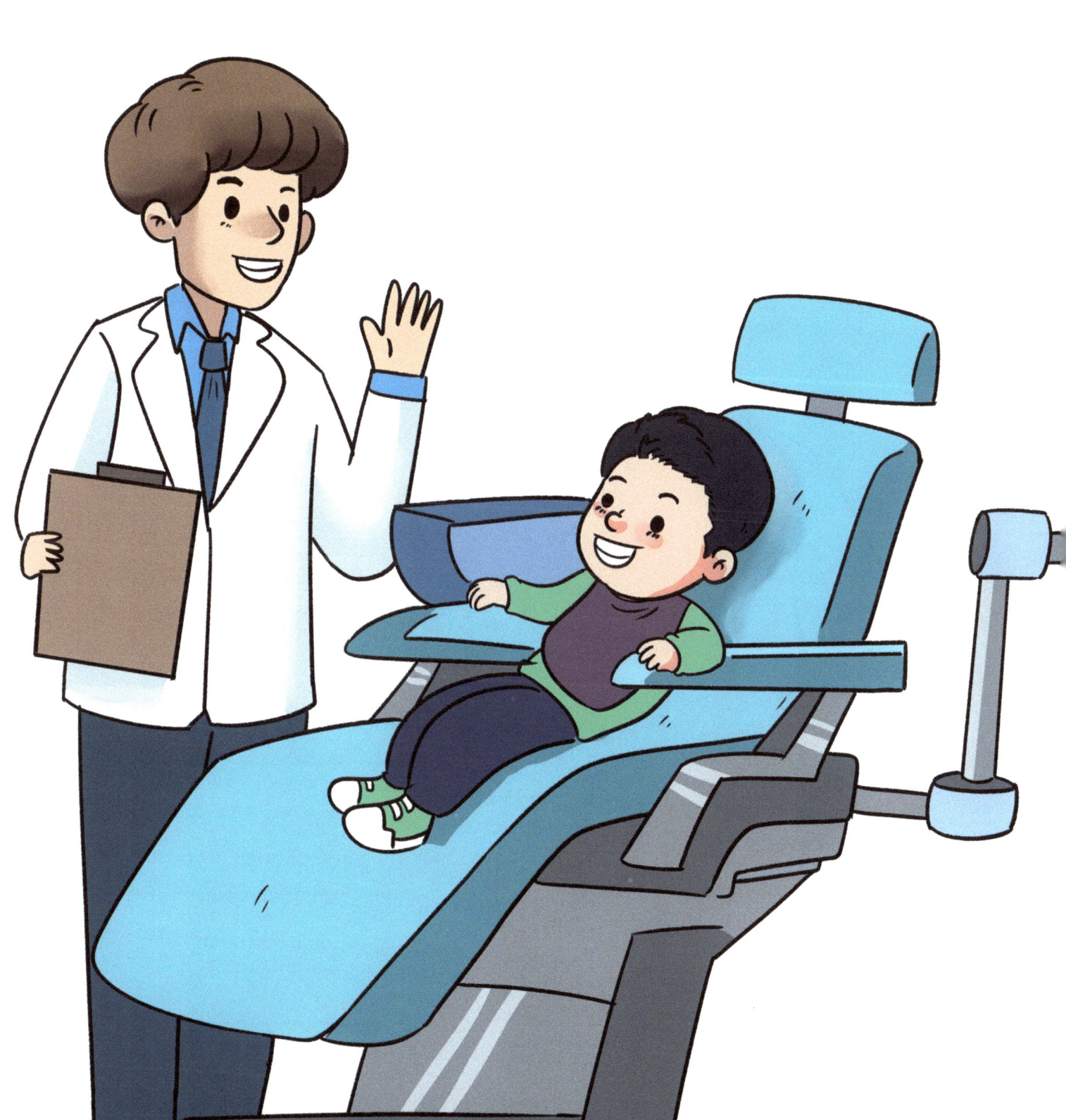

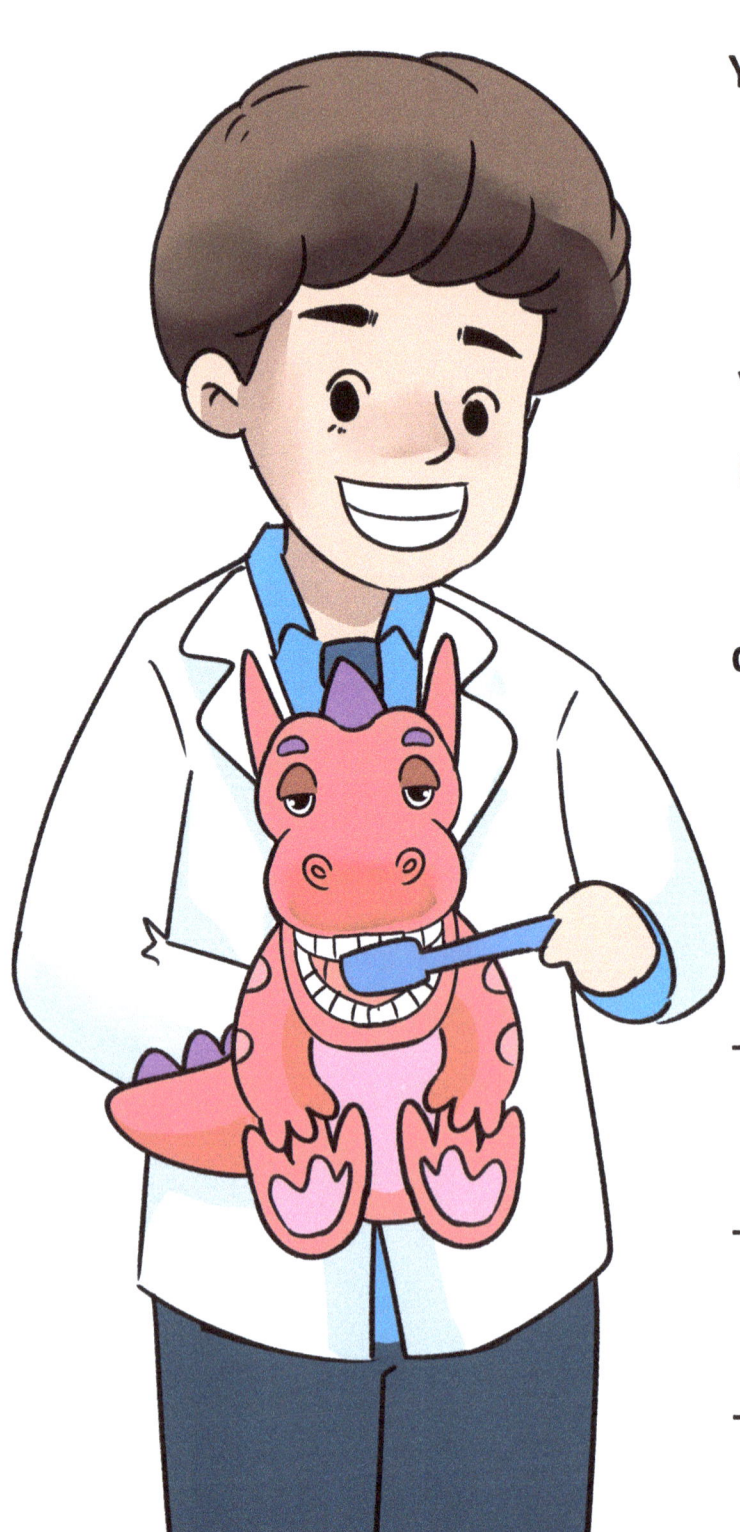

Your dentist will show you how to brush your teeth and use the floss. You will learn how to clean your teeth every day.

If you have questions about how to take care of your teeth, don't be afraid to ask.

Write down your questions here:

_____

_____

_____

Do you floss your teeth everyday?

____ YES   ____ NO

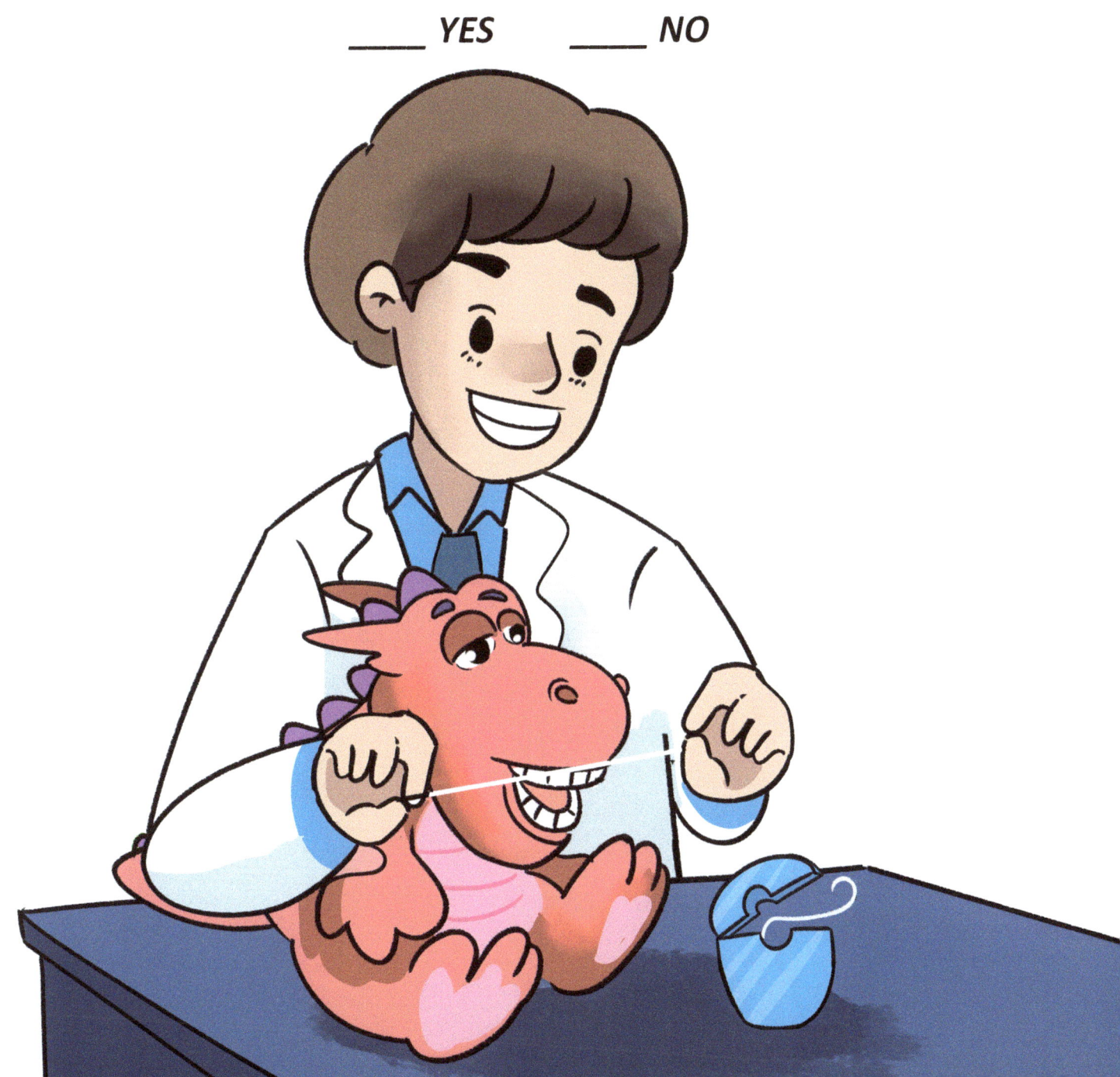

Your dentist will look in your mouth with the bright light to examine your teeth and gums to make sure they stay healthy. They will check for holes in your teeth, known as cavities, caused by sugar bugs eating them.

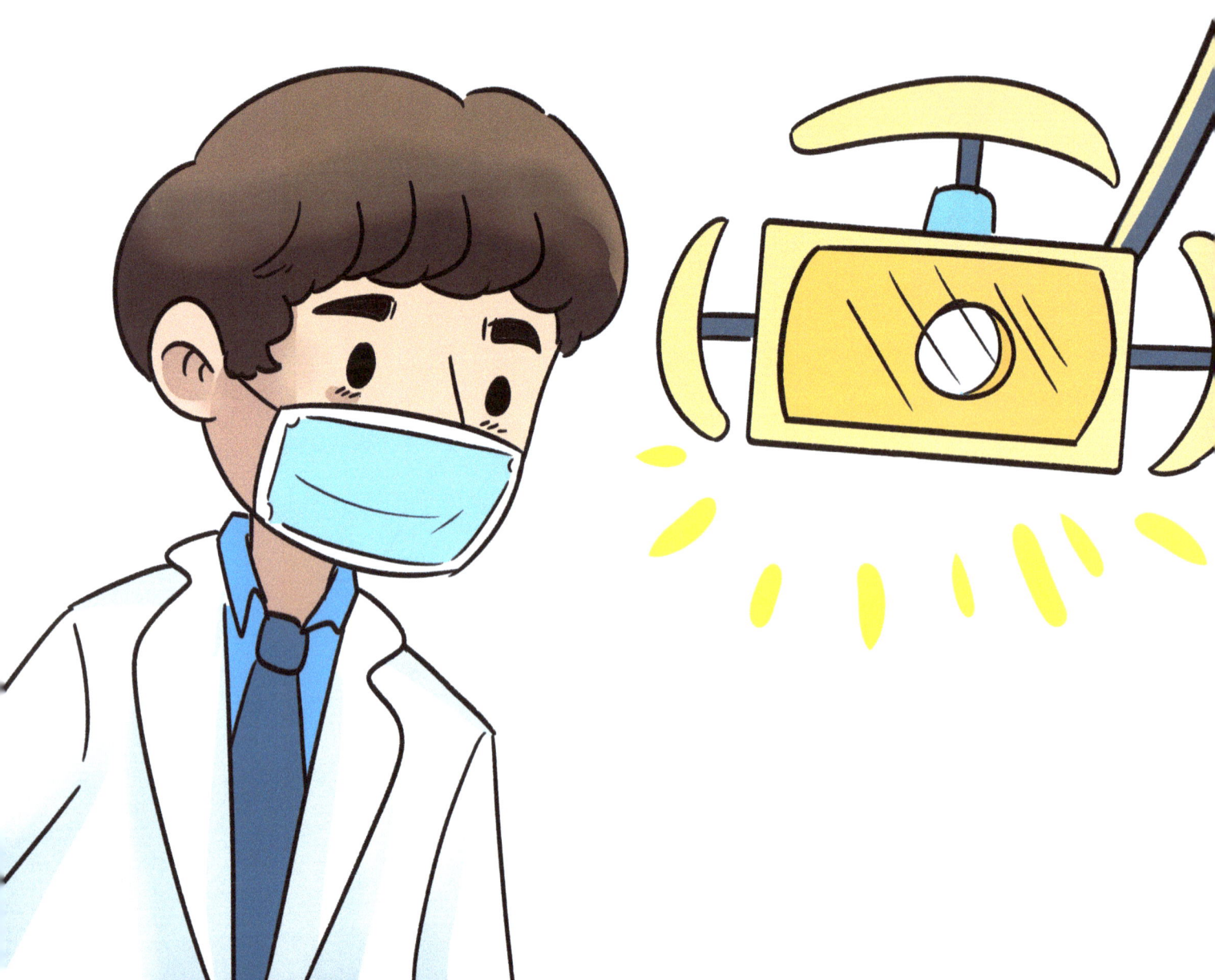

<u>Fun fact</u>: Sugar bugs like to eat your teeth, but you can help stop them by eating less sweets, brushing your teeth 2 times a day (once in the morning and once before bedtime), and flossing everyday.
Brushing your teeth after lunch can also help.

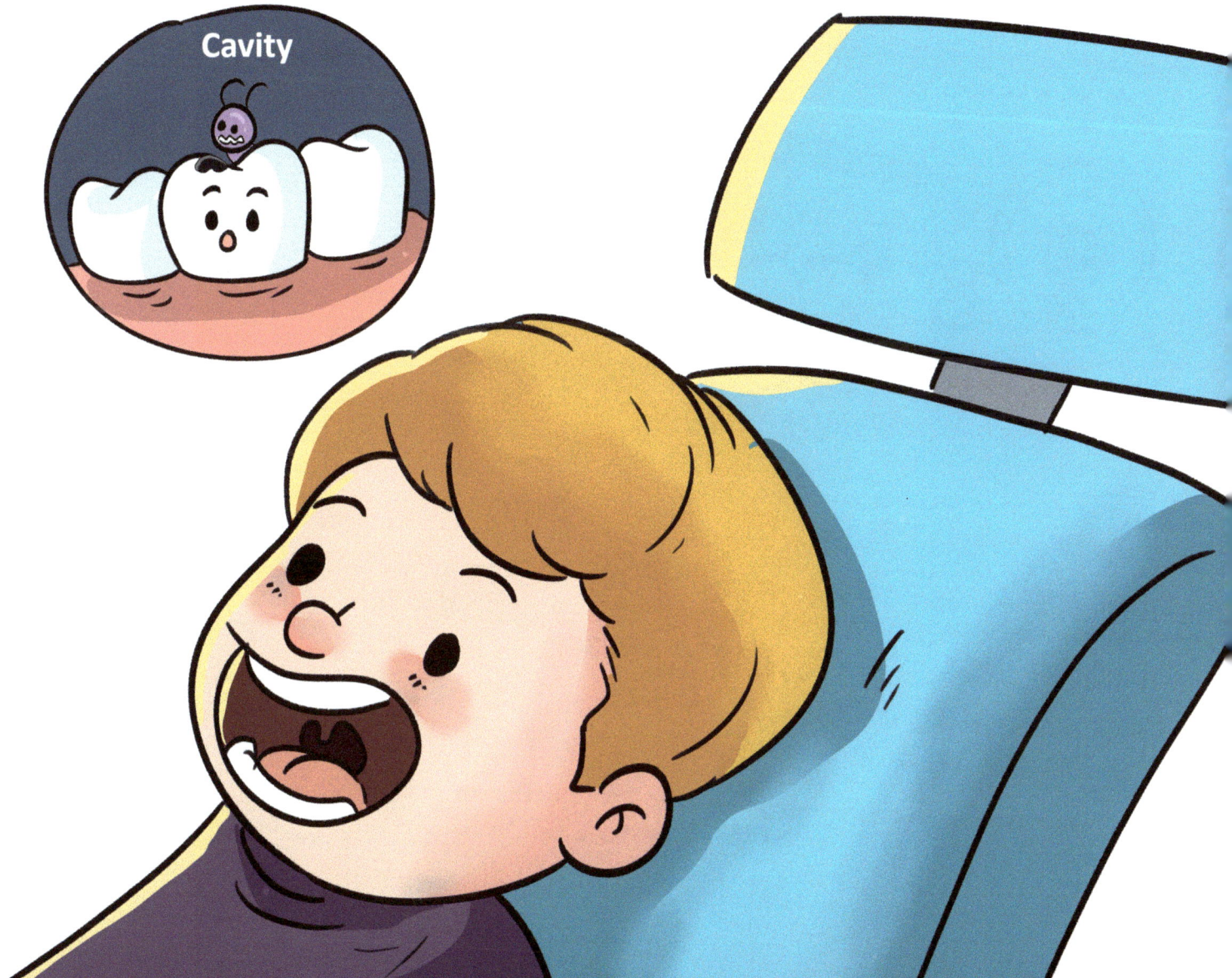

Don't worry. Your dentist will help you clean your teeth.

They may use tools like a small mirror to check your teeth, a tiny water gun that gently sprays water in your mouth, and a little straw-like suction that sucks out the water and the bugs.

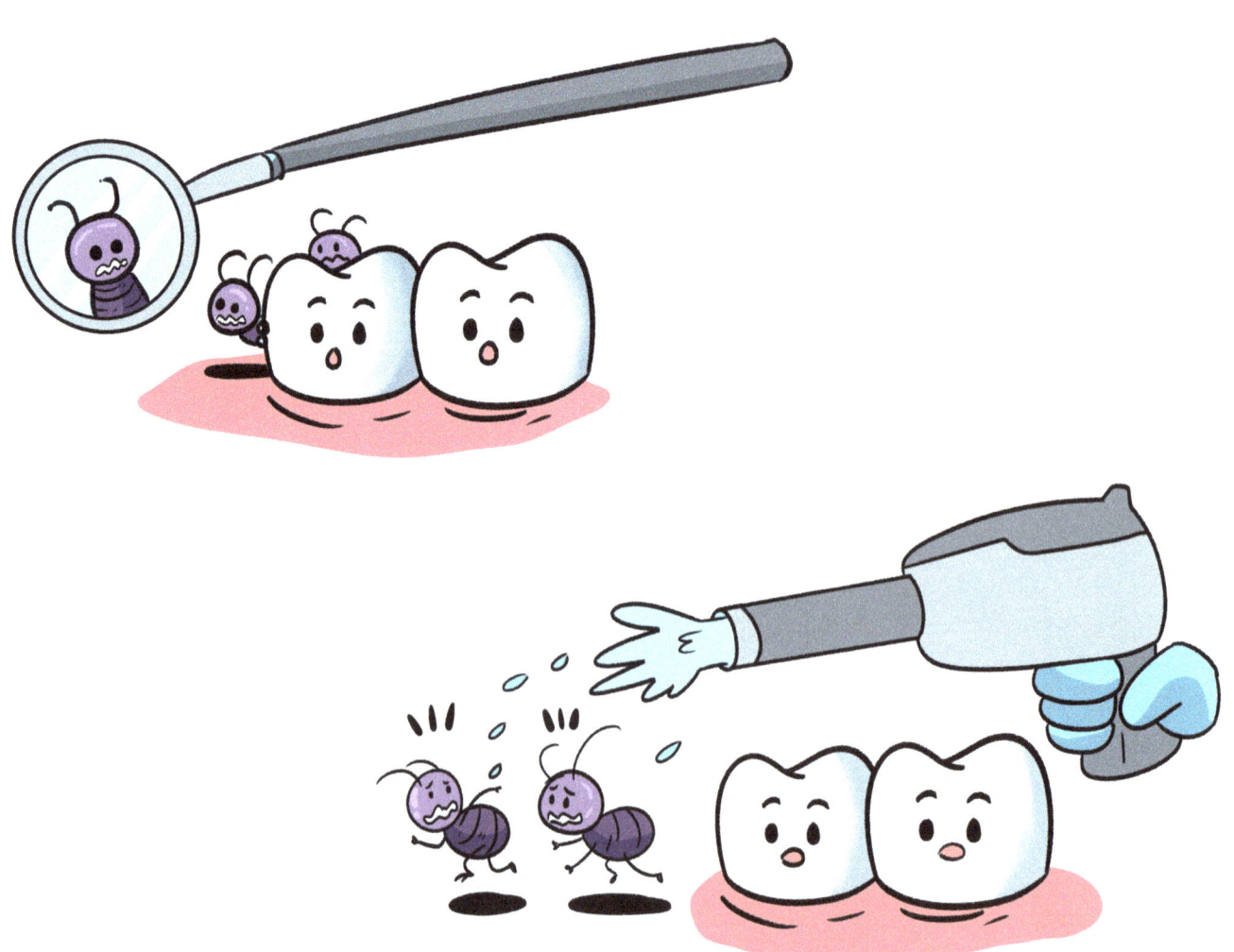

These tools are cool weapons used to keep your teeth clean.

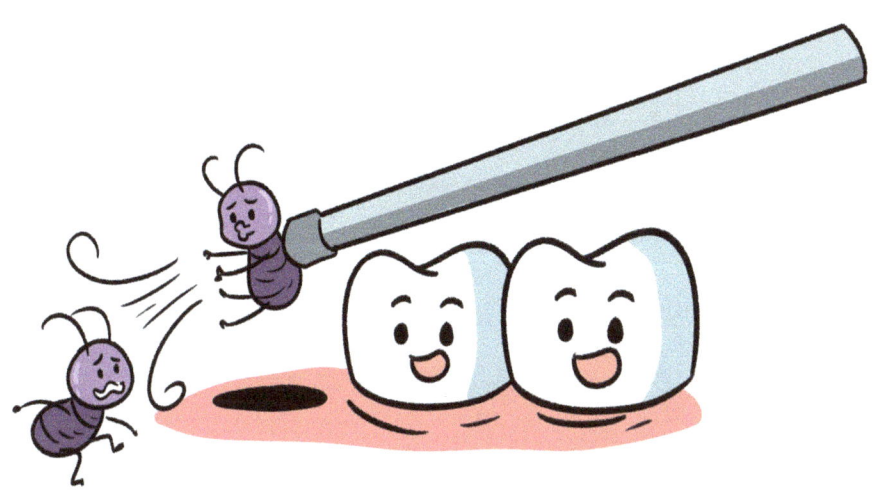

If you have a cavity, your dentist can use a soft-sounding water whistle to help remove the bugs and repair it.

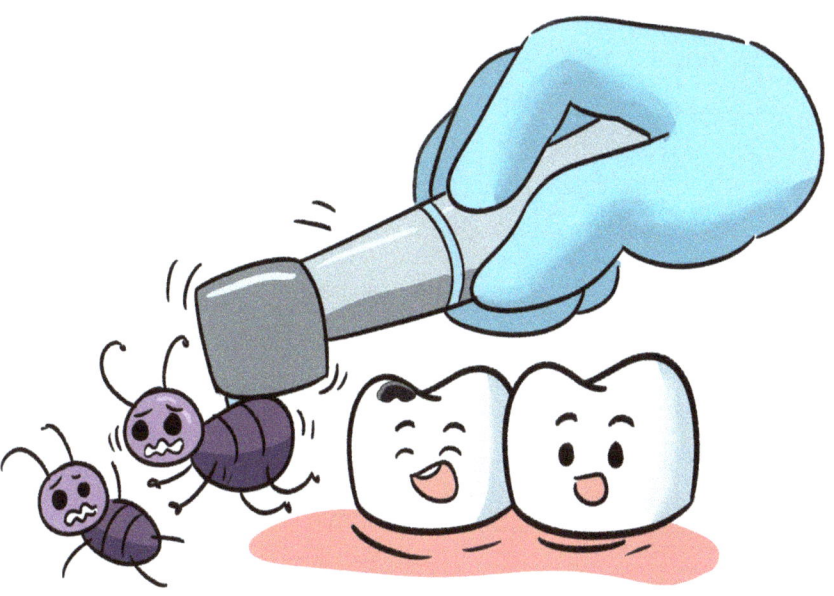

Repairing and filling a cavity can sometimes get tricky because sugar bugs can hide in hard-to-reach spots.

When that happens, you may get some medicine on your gums to make that part of your mouth and tongue sleepy so you don't feel any pain.

The medicine feels like a quick, tiny poke.

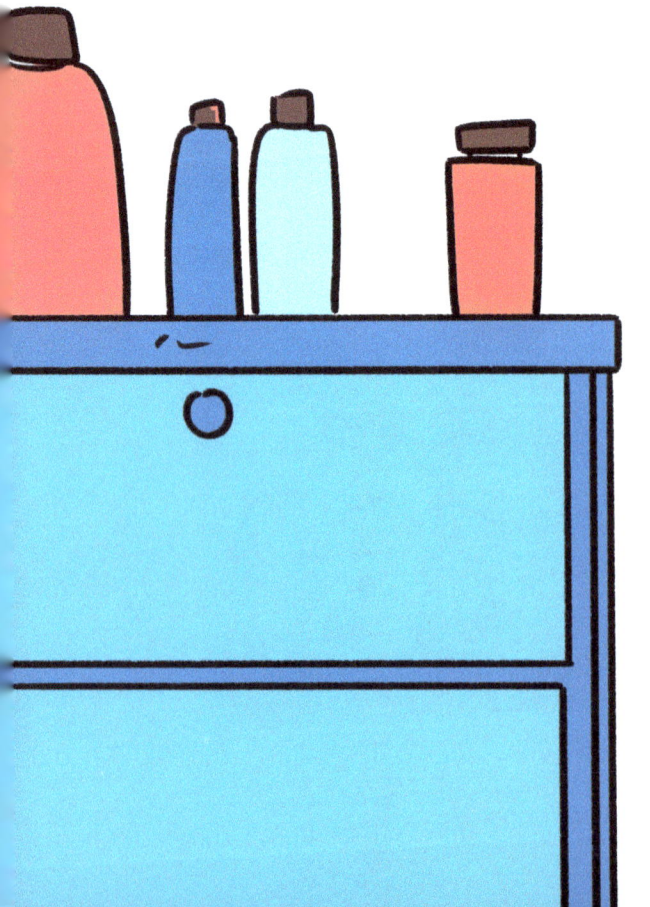

Take a deep breath in (good medicine in) and exhale out (bad bugs out).

You are so brave in this fight against the sugar bugs!

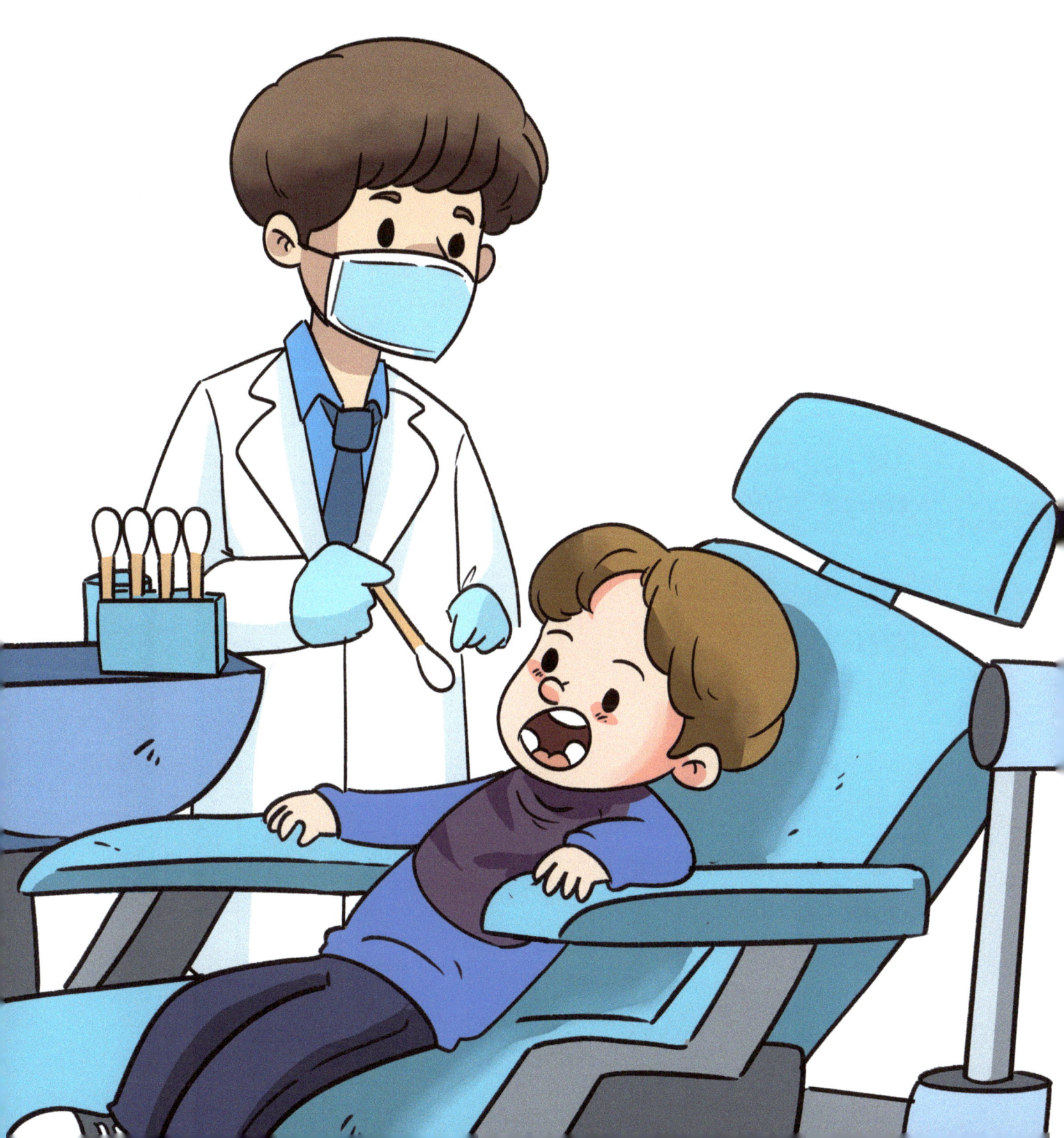

Some kids may need to breathe "laughing gas" to help them relax while their dentist cleans out their cavity and the sugar bugs.

Do you know why it is called "laughing gas?"

Because it makes you **laugh** and feel **silly**, **giggly**, and **relaxed**!

So, if you get laughing gas, don't forget to laugh!

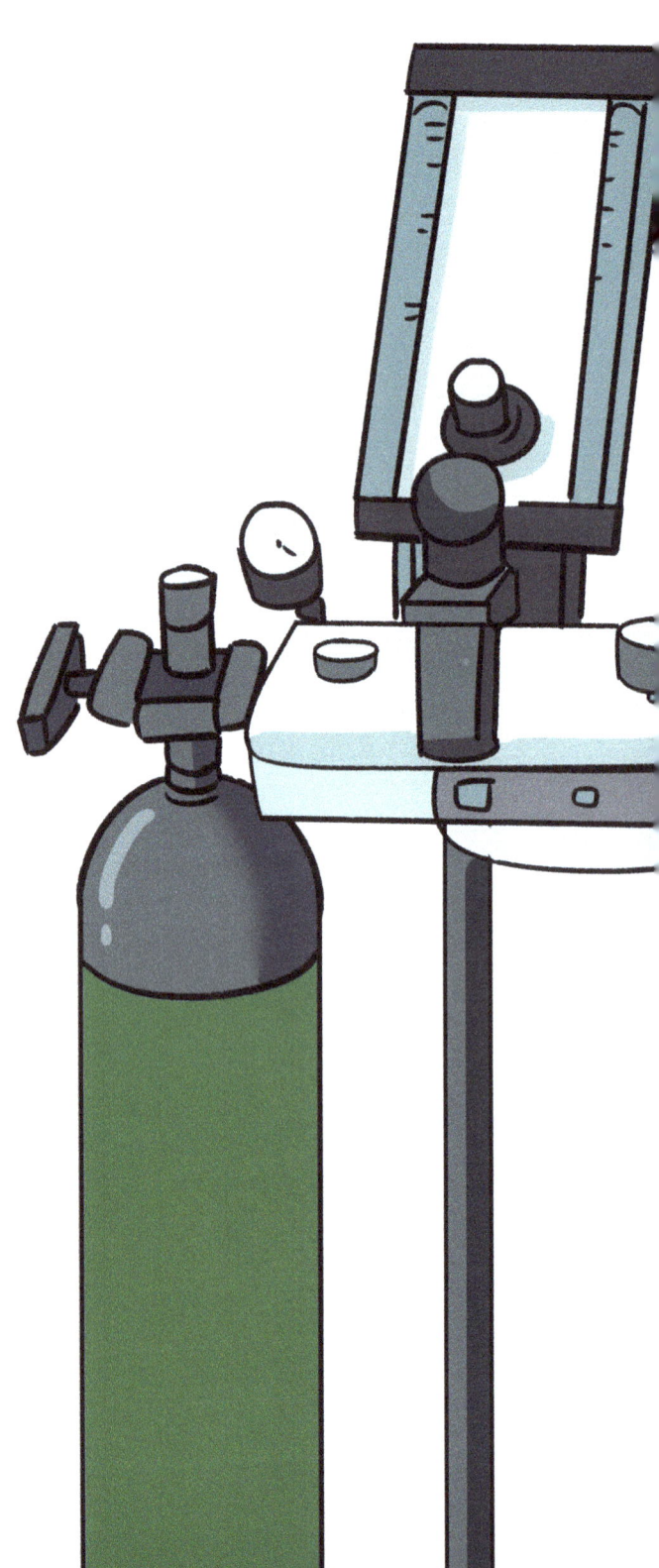

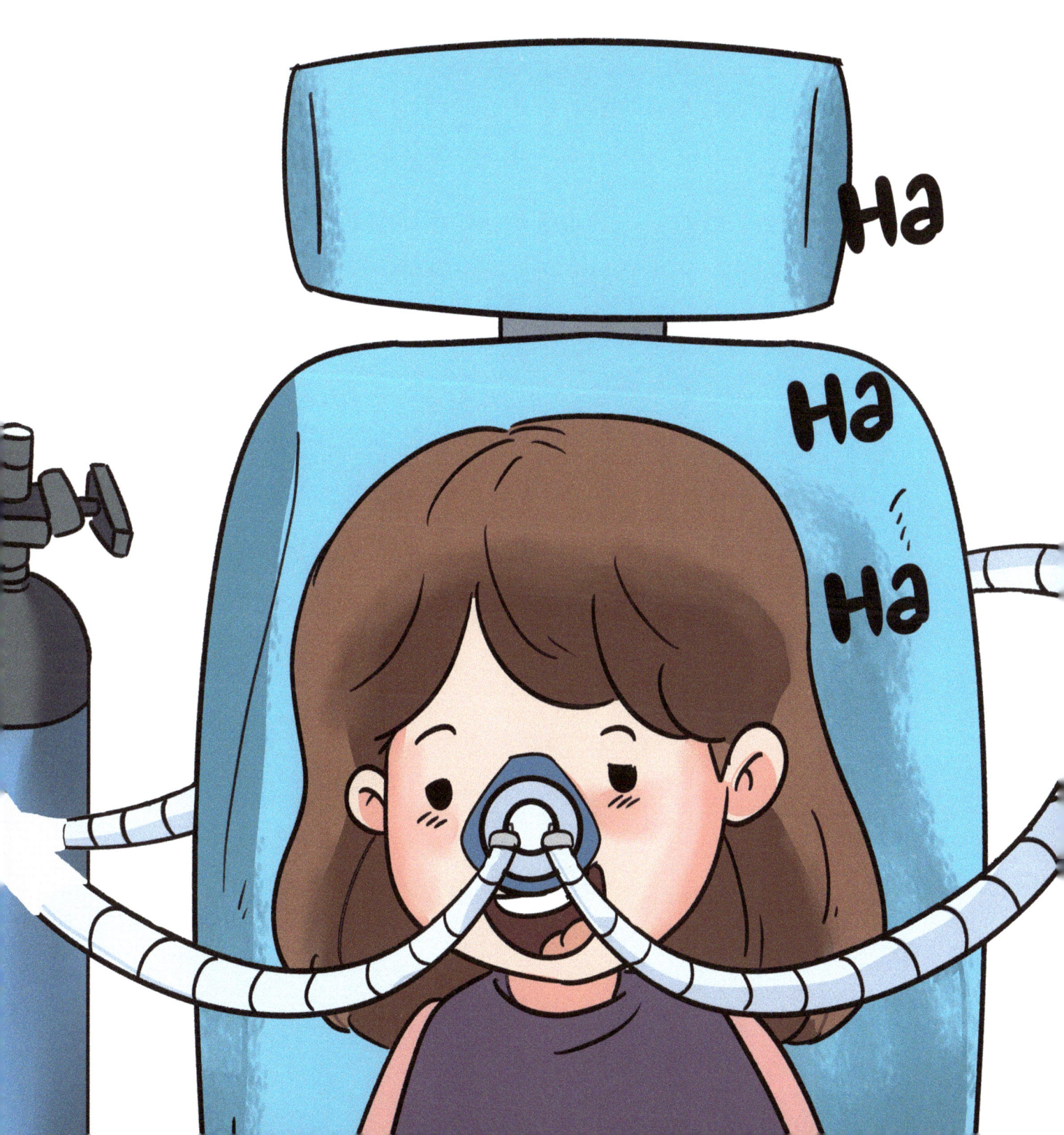

Lastly, they will polish your teeth to make them extra clean and shiny. You then get to rinse your mouth and spit out the water just like when you brush your teeth.

Before you know it, your dentist will be all done. Everyone in the room will see how brave you have been and will be so proud of you!

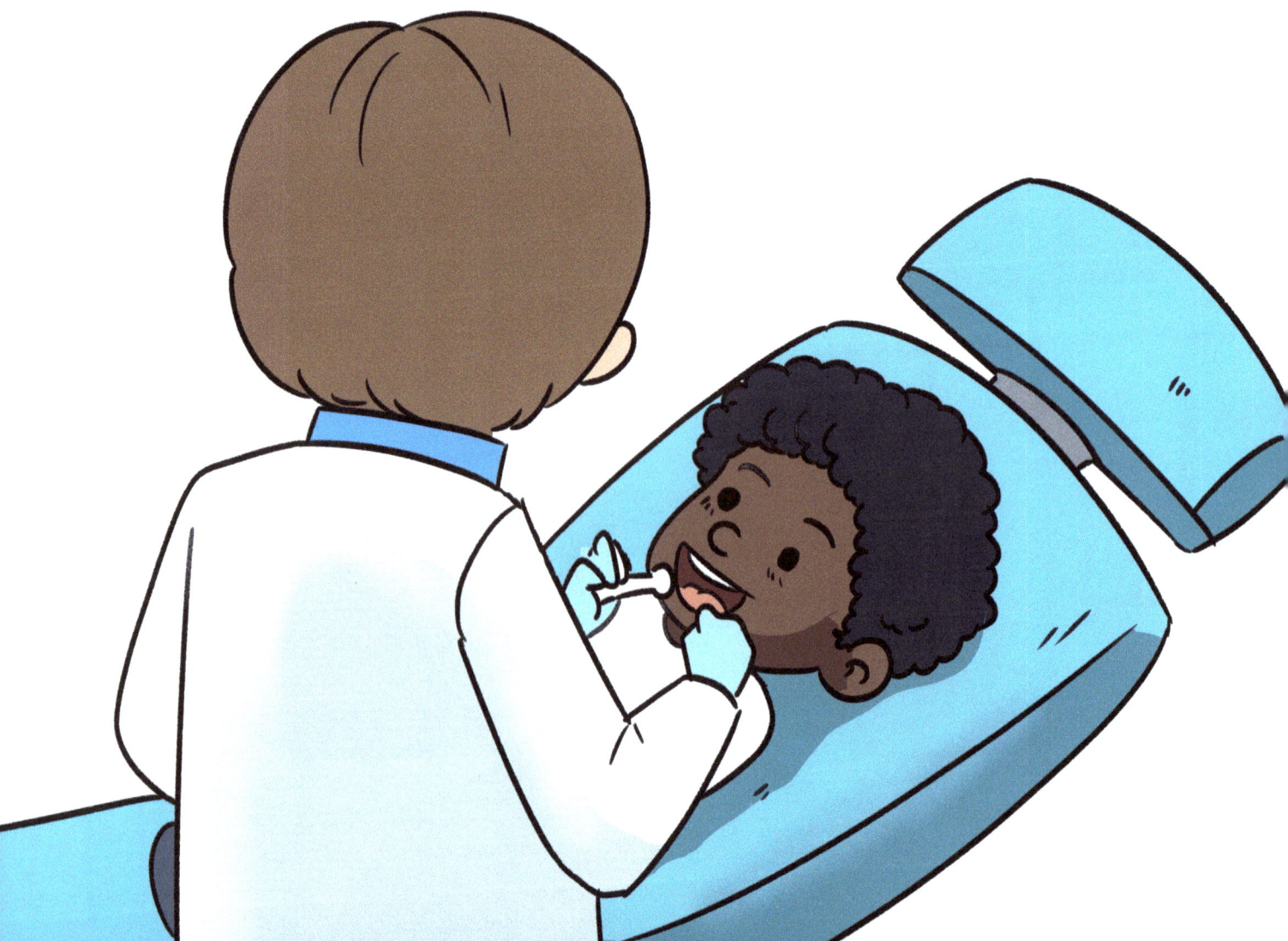

You've done an amazing job, _____!
(Write your name above)

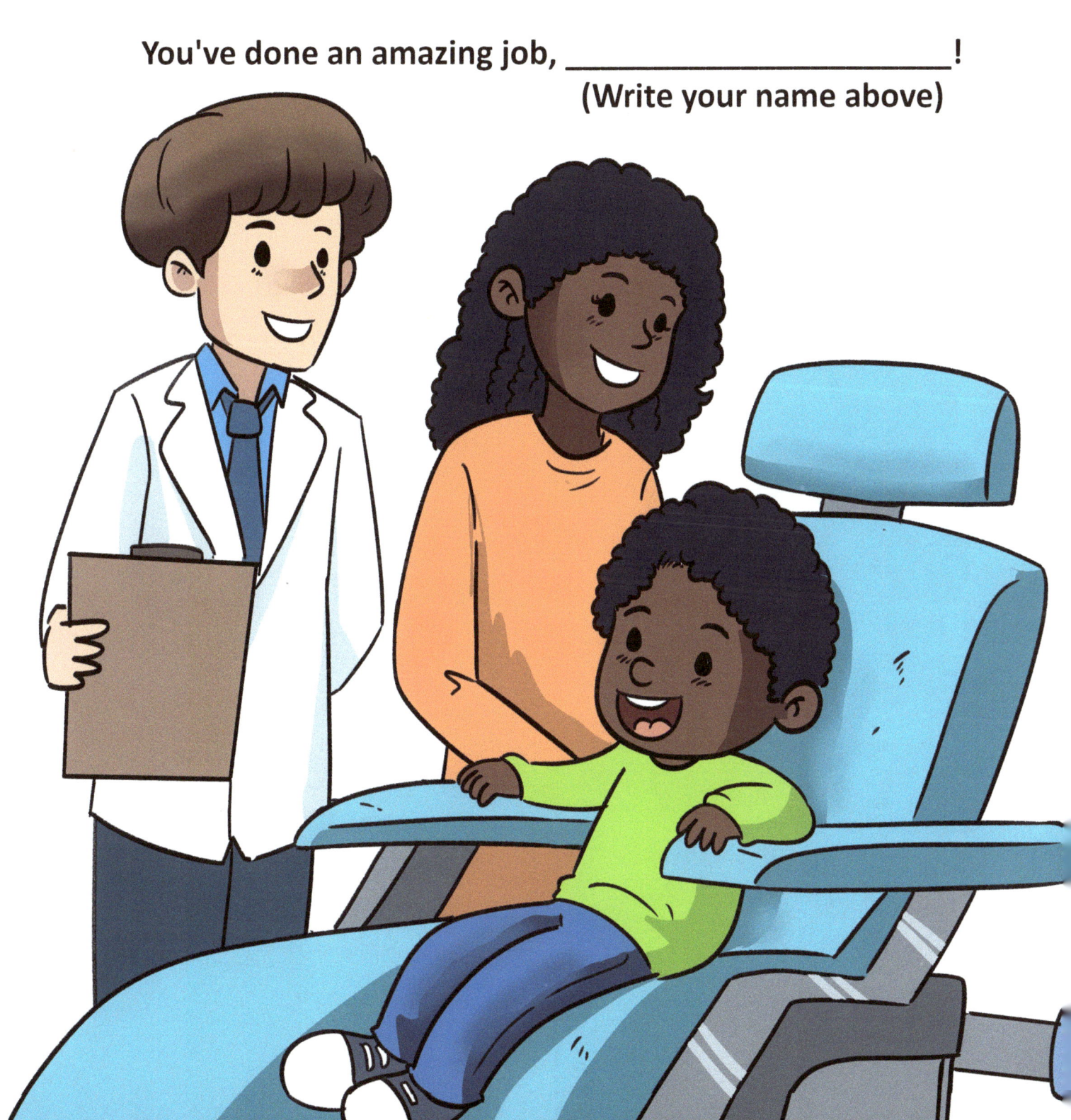

You may not feel your best yet, and that sleepy part of your mouth will take some time to wake up.

So, take it easy and *relax* for now.

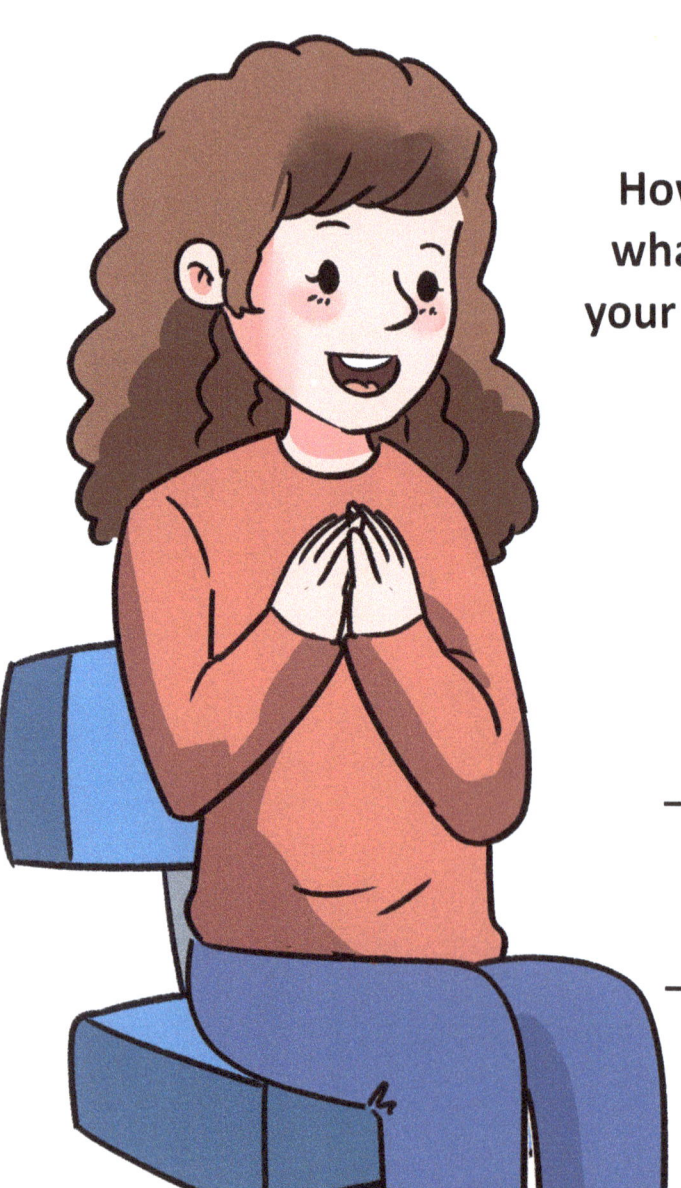

However, you can start planning what you would like to eat when your mouth wakes up from its nap.

Start by making a list here:

_____

_____

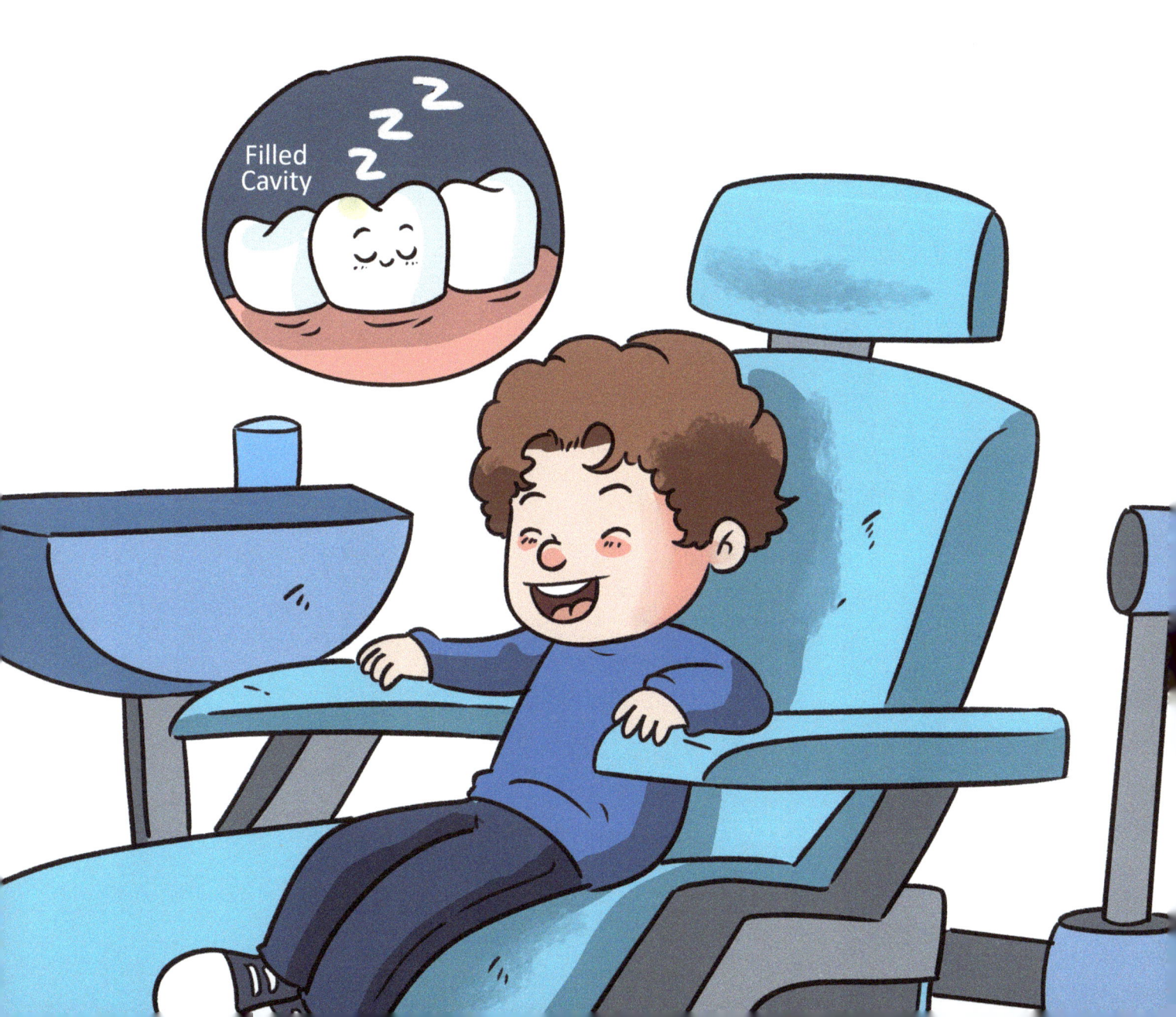

Your adventure at the dentist is almost over.
Before you go home, you will get a brand new toothbrush and toothpaste from your dentist.

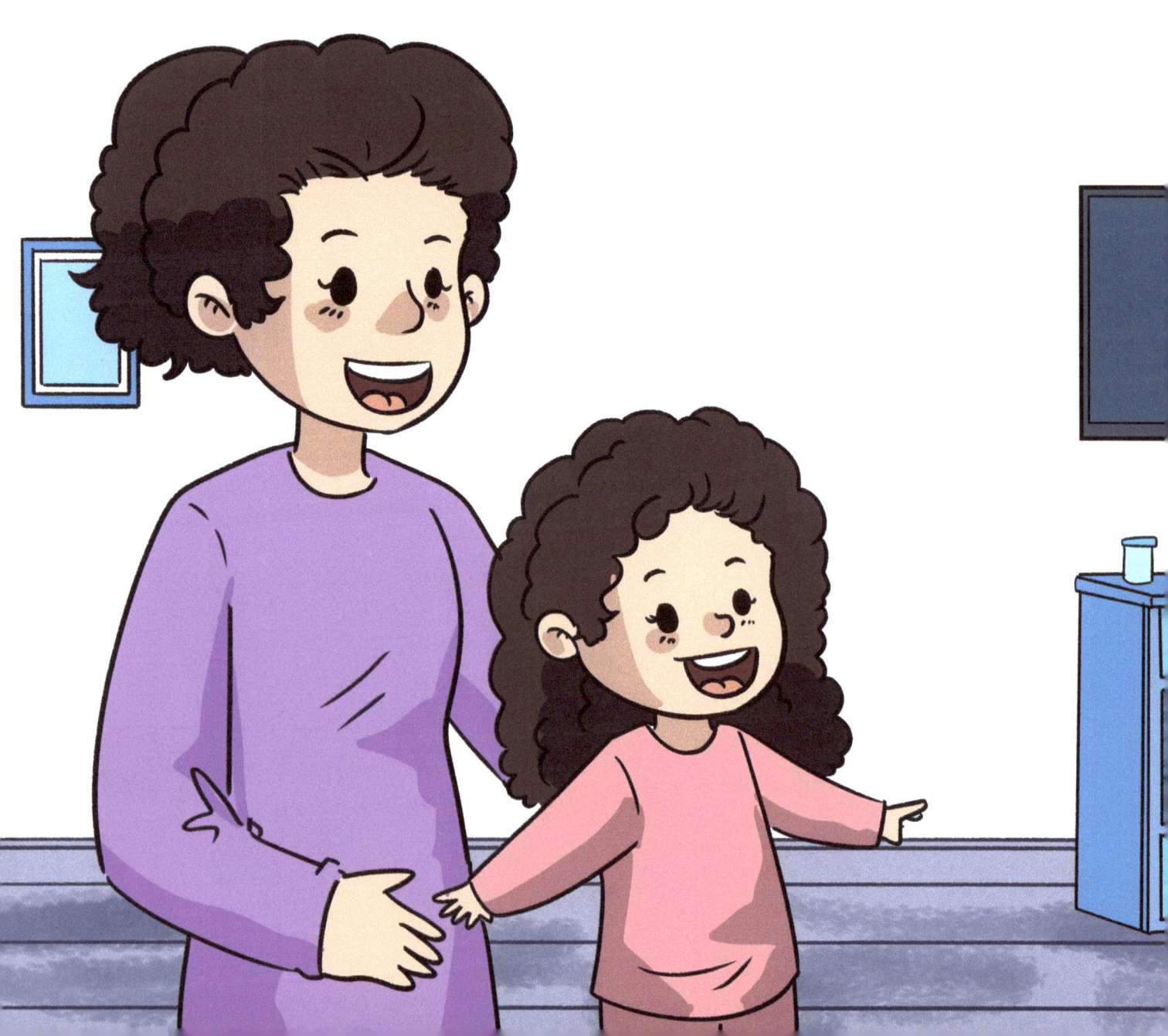

What color toothbrush will you get?
Circle the color of your new toothbrush below.

red   green   yellow   blue   pink   orange   purple

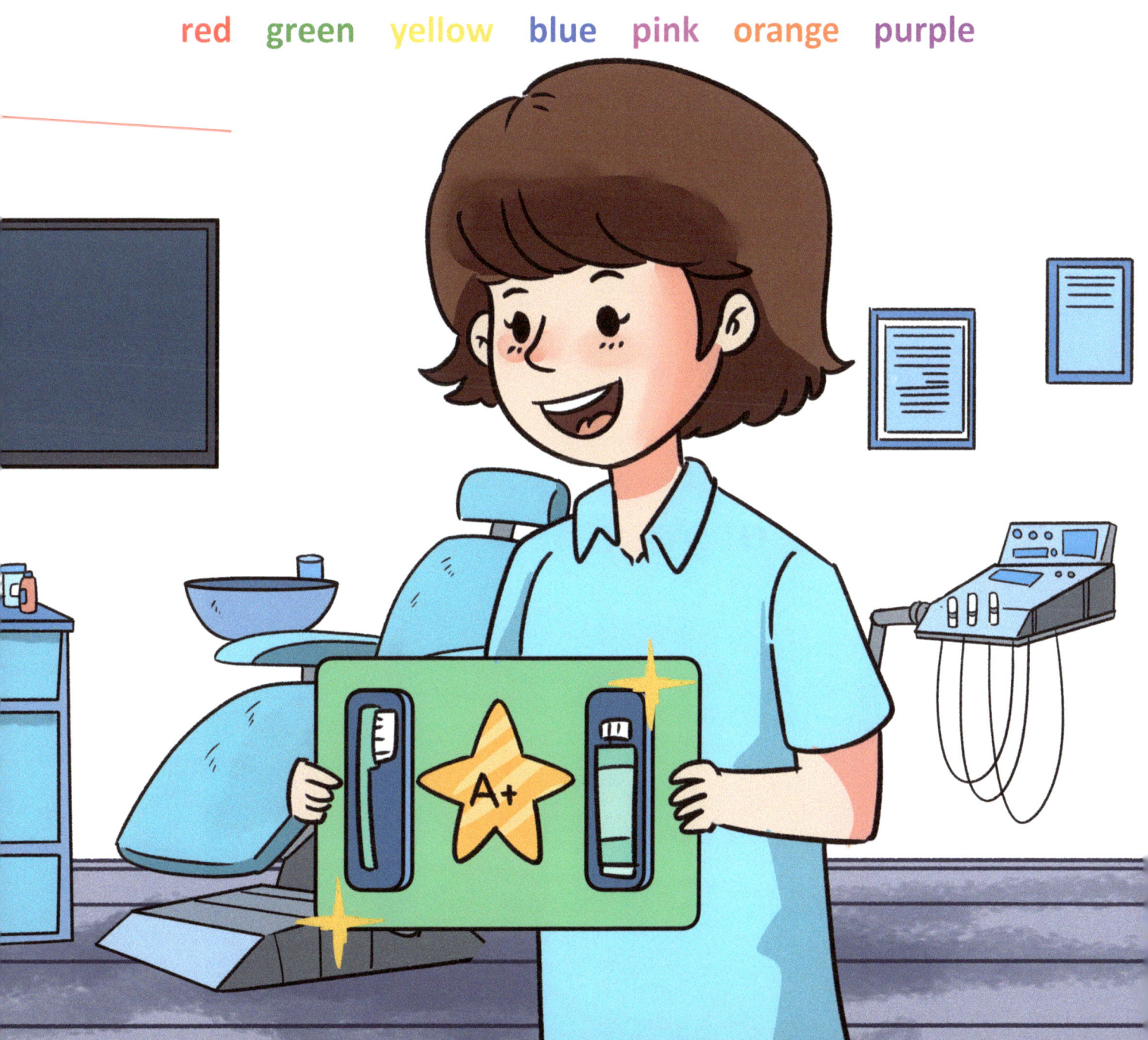

Now that you know how to better take care of your teeth, happy brushing and flossing.

Don't forget to show off your beautiful smile.

See you at your next dentist visit!

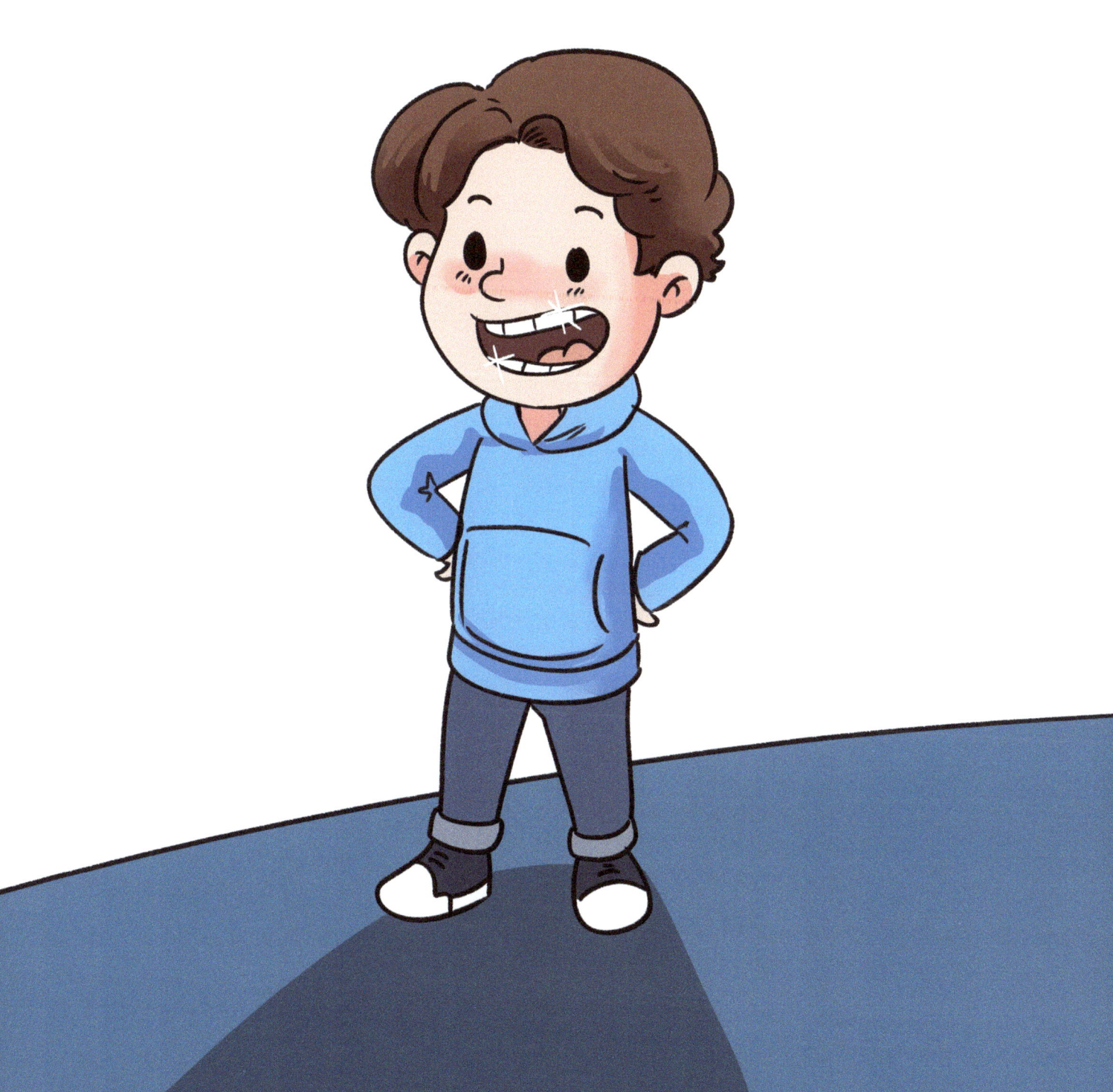

Disclaimer

Please note that the illustrations are not drawn to scale.

This book is written for informational, educational, and personal growth purposes and should not be used as a substitute for medical advice.

Please consult your child's dentist if they need medical attention and to ensure the information in this book pertains to your child's medical condition and needs. I cannot guarantee what your child experiences is exactly what is being discussed in this book.

The author and the publisher are not responsible, either directly or indirectly, for any damages, monetary losses, or reparations due to information in this book. By reading this book, the readers agree not to hold the author and the publisher responsible for any losses as a result of any errors, inaccuracies, or omissions in this book.

Please keep in mind that your child's experience depends on the location, the facility, their medical condition, and the healthcare team. Please use this book in conjunction with your child's dentist's advice. Thank you.

Did this picture book help your child in some way?
If so, I would love to hear about it!

www.amazon.com/gp/product-review/B0DBQ3WM96

For other book titles, please visit:

www.fzwbooks.com

Connect with the author

email: books@fzwbooks.com
facebook/instagram: @FZWbooks

About the Author

Dr. Fei Zheng-Ward is a clinical anesthesiologist who understands the apprehension patients (both adults and children) may have surrounding their upcoming surgery. Her goal in her medical books is to bring useful information to patients so they have a better understanding and appreciation of what happens leading up to, during, and after surgery. She wants readers to be more empowered to make informed decisions and to feel more at ease with their surgery.

As a practicing physician, she takes pride in being respected for her attention to detail, commitment to providing compassionate and personalized patient care, and strong presence in patient advocacy in the perioperative period for each of her patients. She understands the importance of physical and emotional well-being and advocates for patient autonomy.

Her other children's books aim to bring laughter into your family, encourage children to be more helpful at home, and inspire a love of reading.

She is an award-winning author for her book titled ***What to Expect and How to Prepare for Your Surgery***.

More about Dr. Fei Zheng-Ward:

- Board Certified Anesthesiologist

- Anesthesiology Residency Training at The Johns Hopkins Hospital in Baltimore, MD

- Master in Public Health (MPH) degree from Dartmouth Medical School in Hanover, NH

Books by the author

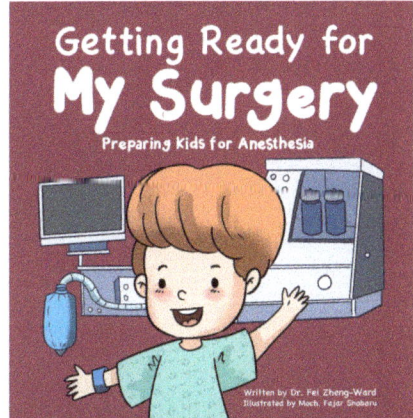
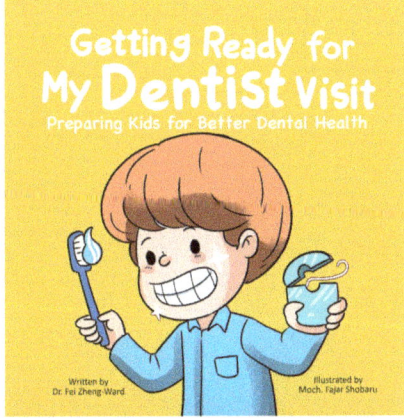
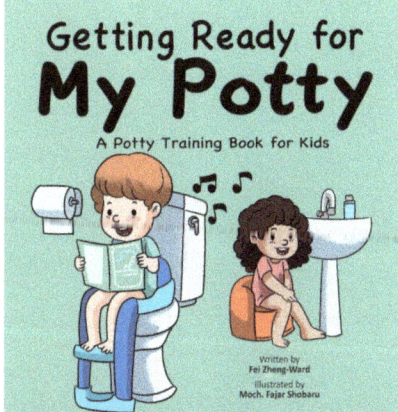
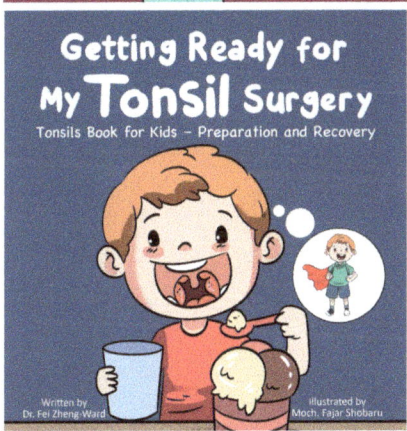
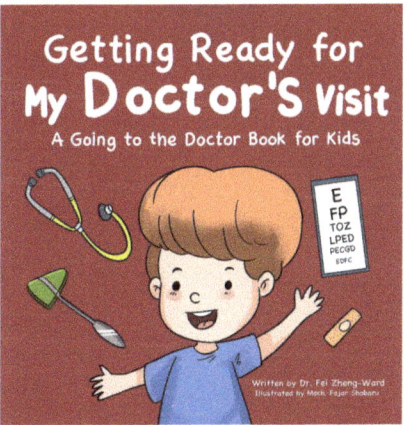
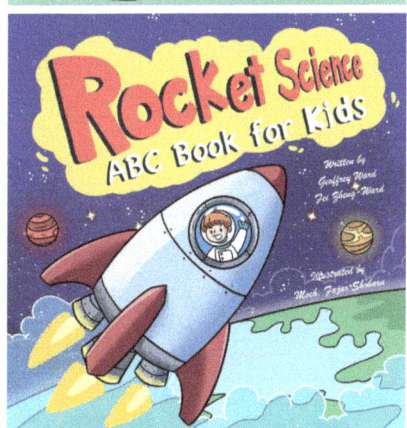
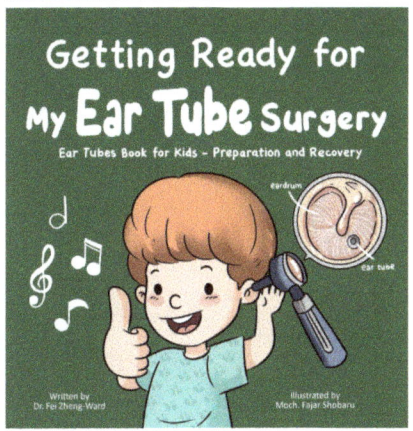
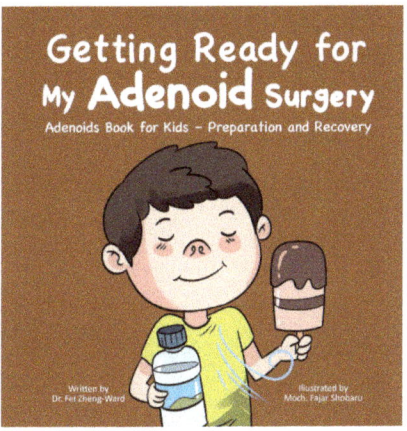
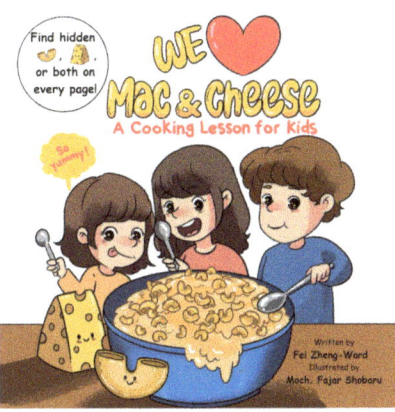

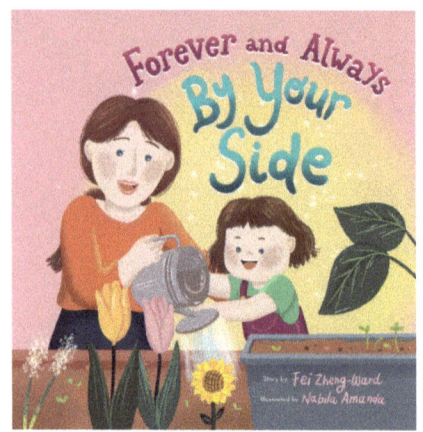
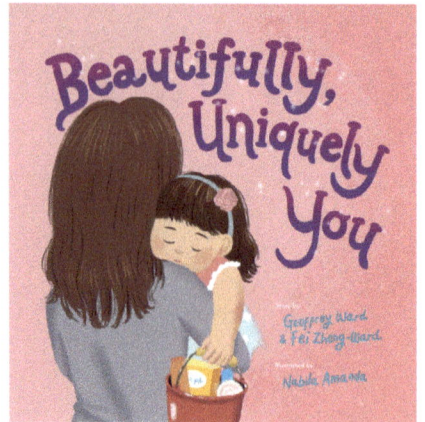
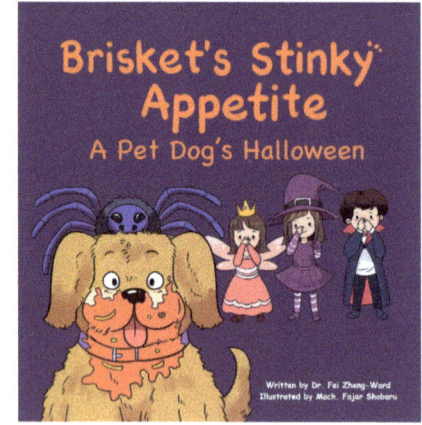
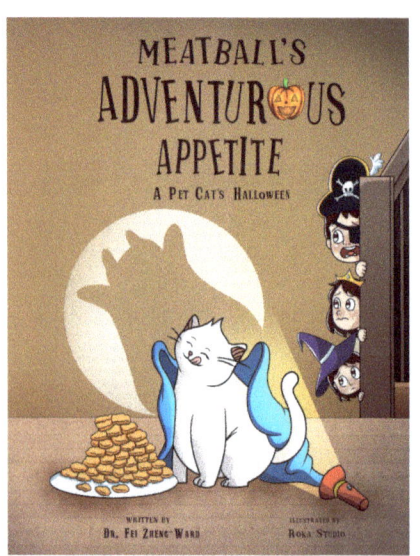
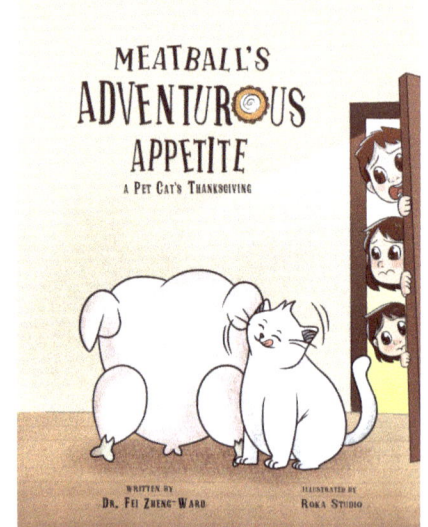
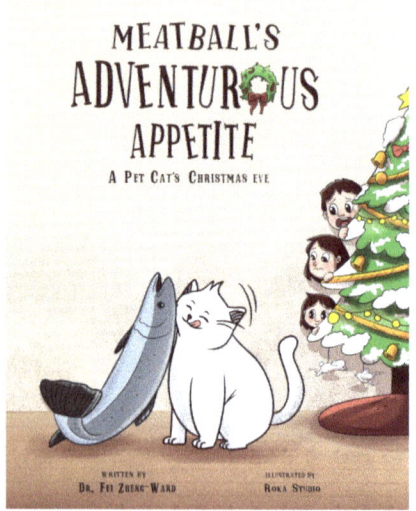
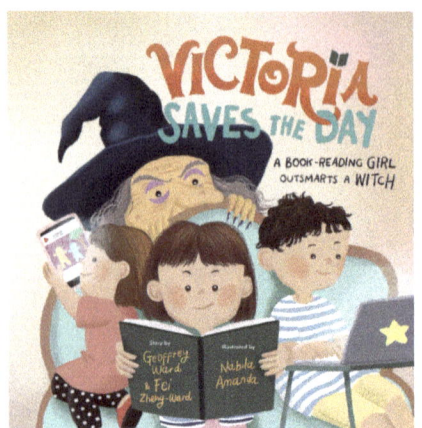
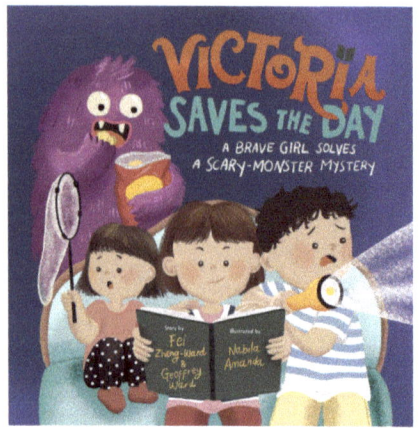
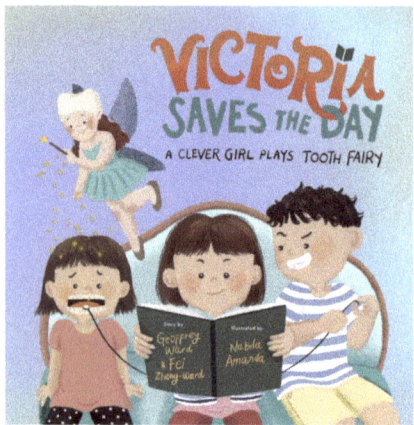

www.ingramcontent.com/pod-product-compliance
Lightning Source LLC
Chambersburg PA
CBHW042359030426
42337CB00032B/5161